INTENSIVE DIABETES MANAGEMENT

SEVENTH EDITION

Edited by
Devin Steenkamp, MD

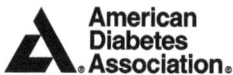

American Diabetes Association.

Director, Book Publishing, Victor Van Beuren; *Managing Editor,* John Clark; *Composition,* Absolute Service, Inc.; *Printer,* Versa Press

Printed in the United States of America
1 3 5 7 9 10 8 6 4 2

The suggestions and information contained in this publication are generally consistent with the *Standards of Medical Care in Diabetes* and other policies of the American Diabetes Association, but they do not represent the policy or position of the Association or any of its boards or committees. Reasonable steps have been taken to ensure the accuracy of the information presented. However, the American Diabetes Association cannot ensure the safety or efficacy of any product or service described in this publication. Individuals are advised to consult a physician or other appropriate health care professional before undertaking any diet or exercise program or taking any medication referred to in this publication. Professionals must use and apply their own professional judgment, experience, and training and should not rely solely on the information contained in this publication before prescribing any diet, exercise, or medication. The American Diabetes Association—its officers, directors, employees, volunteers, and members—assumes no responsibility or liability for personal or other injury, loss, or damage that may result from the suggestions or information in this publication.

⊚ The paper in this publication meets the requirements of the ANSI Standard Z39.48-1992 (permanence of paper).

ADA titles may be purchased for business or promotional use or for special sales. To purchase more than 50 copies of this book at a discount, or for custom editions of this book with your logo, contact the American Diabetes Association at the address below, at booksales@diabetes.org, or by calling 703-299-2046.

American Diabetes Association
2451 Crystal Drive, Suite 900
Arlington, Virginia 22202

DOI: 10.2337/9781580407694

Library of Congress Control Number: 2021939054

Contents

Contributors to the Seventh Edition

Sara Alexanian, MD
Director of Inpatient Diabetes
Clinical Associate Professor of Medicine
Section of Endocrinology, Diabetes and
    Nutrition
Boston University School of Medicine
    and Boston Medical Center

**Megan Bergstrom, PharmD, BCACP,
    CDCES**
Clinical Pharmacy Specialist and
    Certified Diabetes Care and
    Education Specialist
Boston Medical Center

**Kyle Bertram, PharmD, BCACP,
    CDCES**
Clinical Pharmacy Specialist and
    Certified Diabetes Care and
    Education Specialist
Boston Medical Center

Liana Billings, MD, MMSc
Vice Chair of Research and Education,
    Department of Medicine
NorthShore University Health System

Director of Clinical and Translational
    Research and Precision Medicine in
    Diabetes and Metabolism
Clinical Associate Professor in Medicine
University of Chicago Pritzker School of
    Medicine

**Elizabeth Brouillard RD, LDN,
    CDCES**
Outpatient Dietitian and Certified
    Diabetes Care and Education
    Specialist
Boston Medical Center

Katherine Modzelewski, MD
Associate Program Director,
    Endocrinology Fellowship Program
Assistant Professor of Medicine
Section of Endocrinology, Diabetes and
    Nutrition
Boston University School of Medicine
    and Boston Medical Center

Ivania Rizo, MD
Director of Outpatient Obesity Medicine
Assistant Professor of Medicine
Section of Endocrinology, Diabetes and
    Nutrition
Boston University School of Medicine
    and Boston Medical Center

Devin Steenkamp, MD
Director of Clinical Diabetes
Assistant Professor of Medicine
Section of Endocrinology, Diabetes and
    Nutrition
Boston University School of Medicine
    and Boston Medical Center

Catherine Sullivan, MD
Assistant Professor of Medicine
Section of Endocrinology, Diabetes and
    Nutrition
Boston University School of Medicine
    and Boston Medical Center

Elena Toschi, MD
Staff Physician
Joslin Adult Clinic

Director of the Young Adult Program
Assistant Professor
Harvard Medical School

Rationale for and Physiological Basis of Intensive Diabetes Management

Highlights
Rationale for and
Physiological Basis of
Intensive Diabetes Management

- Technological and pharmacological innovations have made it possible for individuals with diabetes to achieve near-normal glycemic control.

- The goal of intensive diabetes management is to achieve near-normal glycemia while minimizing hypoglycemia. This mode of treatment has been supported by large prospective randomized studies as the preferred approach for many patients, with both type 1 and type 2 diabetes, to delay the onset and progression of albuminuria.

- Glycemic control that approaches the nondiabetic state postpones or slows the progression of the retinal, renal, and neurological complications of diabetes.

- Glycemic control that approaches the nondiabetic state improves risk factors that promote macrovascular disease (e.g., plasminogen activator inhibitor-1 levels; platelet aggregation; small, dense low-density lipoprotein cholesterol particles).

- Intensive diabetes management is successful when insulin is delivered and adjusted in amounts required by changes in nutritional intake (e.g., amounts of carbohydrate, protein, fat), physical activity, and various stressors. Successful management of these inter-related issues aims to approximate normal homeostatic fuel metabolism.

- Self-monitoring of blood glucose and/or consistent use of continuous glucose monitoring is essential to guide adjustments in insulin dosage in relation to food consumption and, especially, carbohydrate intake, variation in physical activity, and ambient blood glucose levels to achieve

  - a relatively constant, low plasma insulin level during fasting (postabsorptive state);

  - a rapid increase in plasma insulin levels after meals, in an amount appropriate to the amount of food (primarily carbohydrate) eaten; and

  - a decrease in plasma insulin levels especially during and after prolonged, strenuous exercise or when food intake is delayed.

Rationale for and Physiological Basis of Intensive Diabetes Management

Intensive diabetes management aims to achieve near-normal glycemic control to delay, prevent, or ameliorate diabetes complications.[1] The effectiveness of glycemic control in reducing the risk of microvascular and neuropathic complications is well established.[2,3] Technical advances such as self-monitoring of blood glucose (SMBG), the measurement of glycated hemoglobin A_{1c} (A1C), continuous glucose monitoring (CGM), insulin analogs, and the availability of technically advanced insulin pumps have provided the tools for successful intensive diabetes management.[4,5]

Studies in type 1 diabetes (T1D), in type 2 diabetes (T2D), and in pregnant women with diabetes have shown sufficient benefits to prove the value of intensive glycemic control as a part of the standard of care.[6-8] The landmark Diabetes Control and Complications Trial (DCCT) showed that glycemic control (achieving mean A1C of 7.1%) postpones, prevents, or slows the progression of retinal, renal, and neurological complications.[2,6,9] Follow-up of the DCCT cohort in the Epidemiology of Diabetes Interventions and Complications (EDIC) study has shown persistence of the beneficial effects in the intensively treated subjects even though their glycemic control during follow-up has been equivalent to that of subjects in the conventional treatment arm of the DCCT.[3,10] Glucose lowering in the intensive treatment arm also was associated with long-term benefit with regard to cardiovascular complications, although no magnitude of benefit was shown with regard to cardiovascular mortality.[11-13] Intensive treatment, therefore, should be considered and started as soon as is safely possible after the onset of T1D and maintained thereafter aiming for a target A1C level of ≤7.0%, provided that this can be achieved safely and without frequent and severe hypoglycemia.[9]

The term *intensive diabetes management* became popular in the 1990s after completion of the DCCT, which correlated with the publication of the first edition of this book. Intensive diabetes management of this era emphasized the value of basal bolus insulin therapy or continuous subcutaneous insulin infusion therapy, associated with frequent SMBG and a multidisciplinary team to achieve close scrutiny of blood glucose levels. The approach was most often associated with the care of highly motivated people living with T1D. However, modern intensive diabetes management has evolved and is useful in many people living with T2D, without insulin therapy or frequent SMBG, given the advent of recent potent noninsulin pharmacotherapies and continuous glucose monitoring technologies. This edition continues to recognize the traditional meaning

3

of the term but expands modern principles to a larger group of people living with T1D or T2D with information needed to help each patient move toward treatment goals appropriate for their individual skills and medical condition. The intensive diabetes management approach emphasizes a team approach to patient care.

In T2D, the U.K. Prospective Diabetes Study (UKPDS) in patients with new-onset T2D, and the Kumamoto Study in Japan, similarly, demonstrated significant reductions in microvascular and neuropathic complications with intensive therapy.[14,15] The majority of patients with diabetes succumb to heart attack, stroke, or their consequences. The potential of intensive glycemic control to reduce cardiovascular disease in T2D is supported by epidemiological studies and a meta-analysis.[11] However, three large randomized controlled trials—the Action to Control Cardiovascular Risk in Diabetes (ACCORD), Action in Diabetes and Vascular Disease: Preterax and Diamicron Modified Release Controlled Evaluation (ADVANCE), and Veterans Affairs Diabetes Trial (VADT)—showed that targeting near-normal A1C in high-risk patients with T2D did not have a beneficial effect on cardiovascular disease.[16] Indeed, a treatment strategy designed to lower blood glucose to near-normal levels in the ACCORD trial was associated with increased mortality.[16]

More recently, many antihyperglycemic drugs from the glucagon-like peptide 1 receptor agonist (GLP-1RA) and sodium–glucose cotransporter 2 (SGLT2) inhibitor classes have been shown to improve glycemic outcomes and reduce important macrovascular outcomes, including cardiovascular and all-cause death, stroke, myocardial infarctions, admissions for heart failure exacerbations, and important renal endpoints, including progressive albuminuric diabetic kidney disease and slowed progression toward end-stage renal disease.[17–22] Although an exhaustive discussion of the precise role of these therapies in T2D is beyond the scope of this book, inclusion of one or more of these evidence-based therapies in an intensive diabetes management approach is certainly encouraged.

In addition, aggressive management of blood pressure and lipids, smoking cessation, and antiplatelet therapy are critically important aspects of care, which further reduce the rate of cardiovascular events.[16]

Patients with T1D across the age spectrum, as well as many patients with T2D, adopt intensive management strategies.[9,10,12,13,23] In T2D, this often implies basal-bolus insulin therapy. Indeed, some elderly patients with longstanding T2D experience marked glycemic variability and sensitivity to timing or small differences of insulin doses resembling that of an insulin-deficient patient, and intensive management may be especially appropriate in their care.[16,24–26] Patients with long life expectancy, without advanced diabetes complications or without hypoglycemia unawareness, may benefit from this management strategy.[24,25]

INTENSIVE DIABETES MANAGEMENT

The goal of intensive diabetes management is to achieve near-normal glycemia while minimizing hypoglycemia. Achieving this goal involves the integration of several diabetes treatment components into the individual's lifestyle. These components may include

- an individualized medication regimen;
- frequent blood glucose monitoring;
- CGM;
- the use of pre- and postprandial SMBG data, blood glucose patterns, and trends to meet individually defined treatment goals;
- active adjustment of medication, food, or activity based on glucose measurements;
- active use of carbohydrate counting as a strategy to match food with insulin in patients receiving insulin therapy;
- ongoing interaction between the individual with diabetes and the health-care team;
- assessment, including:
  - education,
  - medical care and treatment,
  - emotional and psychological support, and;
  - frequent objective assessment of glycemic control (A1C- and CGM-derived measurements).

In addition, a thorough understanding of diabetes and its management by all professional personnel involved in the daily care of diabetes is crucial.

Most patients with T1D will require multiple daily insulin injections or an insulin pump to achieve the goals of treatment.[1,4,5] For patients with T2D, successful intensified therapy (with goals similar to those in T1D) may be possible with lifestyle interventions (regular physical exercise and careful medical nutrition therapy to lose weight). In patients with T2D with greater degrees of insulin deficiency, oral glucose-lowering medications (biguanides, sulfonylureas, thiazolidinediones, glinides, α-glucosidase inhibitors, dipeptidyl peptidase-4 inhibitors, SGLT2 inhibitors, and an oral GLP-1RA) given singly or in combination, noninsulin injectable glucose-lowering medications (GLP-1RAs, amylin analogs), or insulin are needed to achieve near-normal glycemia. The goals of therapy should be modified and individualized, taking into account age, comorbid states, ability to adhere to a schedule of regular follow-up assessments, or other individual clinical situations that make the risks of intensified diabetes management greater than the benefits. The balance between risk and benefit may be more delicate in the child without appropriate family support or in the elderly patient.[25]

PHYSIOLOGICAL BASIS OF INTENSIVE MANAGEMENT METHODS

Intensive diabetes management attempts to approximate normal fuel metabolism by delivering insulin or oral diabetes medications to mimic normal glucose homeostatic physiology. Although the goal of completely normal physiology cannot be achieved with available methods, it is possible to improve glycemic control enough to have a dramatic impact on the risk of chronic complications.

NORMAL FUEL METABOLISM

Fuel metabolism is regulated by a complex system involving

- multiple tissues and organs,
- intracellular enzyme systems to use nutrient fuels, and
- hormones and other regulatory factors to
  - distribute ingested nutrients to organs and tissues according to the needs for mechanical or chemical work and tissue growth or renewal,
  - provide storage of excess nutrients as glycogen and fat, and
  - allow release of energy from storage depots as needed during periods of fasting or exercise.

Carbohydrate Metabolism

Glucose is a major energy source for muscles and the brain. The brain is nearly totally dependent on glucose, whereas muscles also use fatty acids and ketone bodies for fuel. The two main sources of circulating glucose are hepatic glucose production and ingested carbohydrate. After absorption of a meal is complete, glucose production by the liver supplies all the glucose needed for tissues such as the brain that do not store glucose. This is referred to as *basal glucose production* and is generally ~2 mg/kg body wt/min in adults. With increasing duration of a fast, as hepatic glycogen stores are exhausted, the relative contribution of gluconeogenesis to basal glucose production increases. Normally ~50% of basal glucose production is from glycogenolysis; the rest is from gluconeogenesis.[27]

Ingested carbohydrates are digested in the intestine into their component monosaccharides. Absorption of glucose causes a postprandial increase in blood glucose level that peaks 60–120 min after the meal. The magnitude and rate of increase in blood glucose are determined by many factors, including the size of the meal, its carbohydrate content, the physical state of the food (e.g., solid, liquid, cooked, raw), the presence of other nutrients (e.g., fat and fiber, which slow digestion), the amount of insulin, and the individual's sensitivity to insulin. The rate of gastric emptying also modulates postprandial blood glucose levels. These factors, in addition to the glycemic index and amount of ingested carbohydrate (together referred to as the *glycemic load*), have significant effects on glycemia.

Glucose is either oxidized for energy or stored as glycogen or fat. After ingestion of oral carbohydrate, 60–70% is stored, mostly as glycogen in liver and skeletal muscle; the remainder is oxidized for immediate energy needs.

Protein Metabolism

Ingested protein is absorbed as amino acids, which may be used in three ways:

1. synthesis of new protein
2. oxidation to provide energy
3. conversion to glucose (gluconeogenesis)

During fasting, proteolysis and conversion of gluconeogenic amino acids to glucose prevent hypoglycemia. Alanine is the major amino acid substrate for hepatic gluconeogenesis; glutamine is the major amino aside substrate for renal gluconeogenesis. Branched-chain amino acids may be used for protein synthesis or oxidized for energy. They are the major donors of amino groups for synthesis of alanine, which can be readily converted to glucose.

Fat Metabolism

Fat is the major form of stored energy. Fat stored as triglyceride is converted to free fatty acids and glycerol by lipolysis. Free fatty acids from adipose tissue may be transported to muscle for oxidation. Oxidation of free fatty acids in the liver produces the ketone bodies acetoacetate and β-hydroxybutyrate (referred to as *ketogenesis*). Synthesis of ketone bodies is, therefore, a stage in fat oxidation; they can be oxidized in extrahepatic tissues to produce energy. Much of the ingested fat in a meal is efficiently stored in adipose tissue or muscle. Normally, only a small fraction of a glucose load is taken up by fat cells. In states of chronic excess nutrition, however, ingested fat is not oxidized and excess nutrients (glucose) are converted to fat and stored in adipose tissue. Elevated circulating free fatty acids from ingested fat or lipolysis blunt peripheral insulin action and slow the postabsorptive decrease in blood glucose.[28]

REGULATION OF FUEL METABOLISM

Fuel metabolism is regulated by several hormones. The central nervous system (CNS) has an important role in this regulation, either through hormones or in other ways that are incompletely understood. The major hormones and their effects are summarized in Table 1.1 and discussed in more detail later in this chapter.

Insulin

Insulin is the major hypoglycemic hormone. It acts on fat and skeletal muscle to increase glucose uptake, oxidation, and storage, and in the liver it stimulates glycogen synthesis and inhibits glucose production. Insulin also inhibits lipolysis and thereby limits the availability of fatty acids for oxidation and inhibits ketogenesis.

Insulin is secreted in two major patterns—basal and prandial. Basal secretion produces relatively constant, low plasma insulin levels that restrain lipolysis and glucose production. Abnormally low levels of basal insulin secretion result in

Table 1.1—Regulation of Fuel Metabolism by Hormones

	Insulin	Glucagon	Catecholamine	Cortisol	Growth hormone
Glucose uptake	+	0	–	–	–
Gluconeogenesis	–	+	+	+	+
Glycogenolysis	–	+	+	+	+
Lipolysis	–	+	+	+	+
Ketogenesis	–	+	+	+	+

+, increases; –, decreases; 0, no effect.

markedly increased glucose production, lipolysis, and ketogenesis, causing hyperglycemia, hyper-fatty acidemia, and ketosis. During exercise, skeletal muscle and other tissues require access to stored energy. Insulin secretion decreases to make stored energy available by allowing increased glucose production and lipolysis to occur. The blood glucose level is the dominant stimulus for insulin secretion. β-Cells of the pancreatic islet constantly monitor glucose levels so that insulin secretion is closely linked to changes in glycemia. Even small increases in blood glucose concentrations normally cause an increase in insulin secretion. Prandial insulin secretion rapidly increases to a level many times greater than basal levels. Higher postprandial insulin levels completely suppress hepatic glucose production and lipolysis and stimulate uptake of ingested glucose by insulin-sensitive tissues.

Counterregulatory Hormones

Glucagon, catecholamines (epinephrine and norepinephrine), cortisol, and growth hormone are termed *counterregulatory hormones* because their actions are opposite to those of insulin. Together with insulin, they regulate metabolism under widely varying conditions. These hormones often are referred to as *stress hormones* because their levels in the circulation increase in response to stress. It has been suggested that this response is designed to provide the extra energy that may be needed to cope with stress. The concept of hypoglycemia-associated autonomic failure (HAAF) in diabetes posits that recent antecedent iatrogenic hypoglycemia causes both defective glucose counterregulation (by reducing the epinephrine response to falling glucose levels in the setting of an absent glucagon response) and hypoglycemia unawareness (by reducing the autonomic and the resulting neurogenic symptom responses) and thus a vicious cycle of recurrent hypoglycemia. Perhaps the most compelling support of HAAF is the finding that as few as 2–3 weeks of avoidance of hypoglycemia reverses hypoglycemia unawareness and improves the reduced epinephrine component of defective glucose counterregulation in most affected individuals.[29]

Glucagon. Glucagon is the first line of defense against hypoglycemia in people who do not have diabetes. When blood glucose levels fall, the plasma glucagon concentration rapidly increases, and glucagon potently and rapidly stimulates hepatic glucose production by increasing glycogenolysis and gluconeogenesis. In T1D, despite the loss of β-cell function, glucagon secretion by the pancreatic α-cells persists. Glucagon secretion can promote hepatic glucogenesis inappropriate to ambient glucose elevations, which in part is responsible for triggering fasting hyperglycemia and mediating the rise of glucose that occurs despite fasting or emesis when insulin levels are insufficient. Conversely, appropriate glucagon responsiveness to hypoglycemia is lost among many people with long-standing diabetes, especially if their diabetes has been tightly controlled, resulting in the loss of this important defense mechanism against hypoglycemia.[29,30]

Catecholamines. Catecholamines are produced at times of stress (fight or flight) and also stimulate the release of stored energy. Epinephrine stimulates glucose production and limits glucose utilization in insulin-sensitive tissues, such as skeletal muscle. Catecholamines are the major defense against hypoglycemia in patients with T1D who have lost their glucagon response to hypoglycemia. Hypoglycemia unawareness and sluggish recovery from hypoglycemia may occur when this defense is defective. Patients with hypoglycemia unawareness are at considerably increased risk for severe and prolonged hypoglycemia, and they should embark on intensified glucose control only with great caution after a period of hypoglycemia avoidance and restoration of catecholamine responsiveness.[29,31]

Cortisol. Secretion of the hormone cortisol also increases at times of stress. Its major effect is to stimulate gluconeogenesis; however, the onset of this effect is much slower than that of glucagon. The hyperglycemic response to cortisol is delayed for several hours. Consequently, cortisol is not effective in protecting against acute hypoglycemia. Cortisol also limits glucose utilization in several tissues including skeletal muscle.[29,32]

Growth hormone. Growth hormone also has slow effects on glucose metabolism. A major surge of growth hormone secretion occurs during sleep and is responsible for an increase in insulin resistance in the early morning, termed the *dawn phenomenon.* Normally, a slight increase in insulin secretion compensates for the effects of nocturnal growth hormone secretion, but in diabetes, the result may be morning hyperglycemia.

IMPLICATIONS FOR THERAPY

The most effective treatment regimens for diabetes attempt to replicate normal physiology. Important elements of treatment include

- a relatively constant low blood insulin level during fasting;
- a rapid increase in blood insulin levels with meals, in an amount appropriate to the quantity and macronutrient content of food eaten;
- a decrease in insulin levels with vigorous and especially prolonged exercise or prolonged fasting; and
- frequent blood glucose measurements and CGM to guide adjustments in insulin dose and other components of the regimen.
  - automation of insulin delivery, relying on insulin pumps equipped with various computerized control algorithms which are, in turn, dependent on real-time CGM data input in appropriate patients with T1D[5]

Even the most complicated regimen cannot account for all the conditions that influence blood glucose levels. Indeed, for patients using insulin, variable absorption of insulin from its subcutaneous injection site is one important factor contributing to blood glucose variation. Therefore, even the best methods currently available do not produce "perfect control." Patients with diabetes may adhere to every aspect of management and still experience unexplained blood glucose variations. These patients should be counseled to expect some variability in blood glucose levels that may be difficult or impossible to account for. Nonetheless, meticulous attention to many small details greatly improves the control that can be achieved.

REFERENCES

1. Ahern JA, Boland EA, Doane R, et al. Insulin pump therapy in pediatrics: a therapeutic alternative to safely lower HbA1c levels across all age groups. *Pediatr Diabetes* 2002;3(1):10–15

2. Nathan DM, Genuth S, Lachin J, et al. The effect of intensive treatment of diabetes on the development and progression of long-term complications in insulin-dependent diabetes mellitus. *N Engl J Med* 1993;329(14):977–986

3. The Diabetes Control and Complications Trial Research Group. Hypoglycemia in the Diabetes Control and Complications Trial. *Diabetes* 1997;46(2):271–286

4. Hirsch IB. Insulin analogues. *N Engl J Med* 2005;352(2):174–183

5. American Diabetes Association. 7. Diabetes technology: *Standards of Medical Care in Diabetes—2020. Diabetes Care* 2020;43(Suppl. 1):S77–S88

6. American Diabetes Association. *Standards of Medical Care in Diabetes—2016* abridged for primary care providers. *Clin Diabetes* 2016;34(1):3–21

7. Kitzmiller JL, Block JM, Brown FM, et al. Managing preexisting diabetes for pregnancy: summary of evidence and consensus recommendations for care. *Diabetes Care* 2008;31(5):1060–1079

8. American Diabetes Association. *Standards of Medical Care in Diabetes—2020* abridged for primary care providers. *Clin Diabetes* 2020;38(1):10–38

9. Writing Team for the Diabetes Control and Complications Trial/Epidemiology of Diabetes Interventions and Complications Research Group. Effect of intensive therapy on the microvascular complications of type 1 diabetes mellitus. *JAMA* 2002;287(19):2563–2569

10. Writing Team for the Diabetes Control and Complications Trial/Epidemiology of Diabetes Interventions and Complications Research Group. Sustained effect of intensive treatment of type 1 diabetes mellitus on development and progression of diabetic nephropathy: the Epidemiology of Diabetes Interventions and Complications (EDIC) study. *JAMA* 2003;290(16):2159–2167

11. Gaede P, Vedel P, Larsen N, et al. Multifactorial intervention and cardiovascular disease in patients with type 2 diabetes. *N Engl J Med* 2003;348(5):383–393

12. Nathan DM, Cleary PA, Backlund JY, et al. Intensive diabetes treatment and cardiovascular disease in patients with type 1 diabetes. *N Engl J Med* 2005;353(25):2643–2653

13. Nathan DM, Lachin J, Cleary P, et al. Intensive diabetes therapy and carotid intima-media thickness in type 1 diabetes mellitus. *N Engl J Med* 2003;348(23):2294–2303

14. Shichiri M, Kishikawa H, Ohkubo Y, Wake N. Long-term results of the Kumamoto Study on optimal diabetes control in type 2 diabetic patients. *Diabetes Care* 2000;23(Suppl. 2):B21–B29

15. Stratton IM, Adler AI, Neil HA, et al. Association of glycaemia with macrovascular and microvascular complications of type 2 diabetes (UKPDS 35): prospective observational study. *BMJ* 2000;321(7258):405–412

16. Skyler JS, Bergenstal R, Bonow RO, et al. Intensive glycemic control and the prevention of cardiovascular events: implications of the ACCORD, ADVANCE, and VA diabetes trials: a position statement of the American Diabetes Association and a scientific statement of the American College of Cardiology Foundation and the American Heart Association. *J Am Coll Cardiol* 2009;53(3):298–304

17. Aroda VR, Ahmann A, Cariou B, et al. Comparative efficacy, safety, and cardiovascular outcomes with once-weekly subcutaneous semaglutide in the treatment of type 2 diabetes: insights from the SUSTAIN 1–7 trials. *Diabetes Metab* 2019;45(5):409–418

18. Sridhar VS, Rahman HU, Cherney DZI. What have we learned about renal protection from the cardiovascular outcome trials and observational analyses with SGLT2 inhibitors? *Diabetes Obes Metab* 2020;22(Suppl. 1):55–68

19. McMurray JJV, Solomon SD, Inzucchi SE, et al. Dapagliflozin in patients with heart failure and reduced ejection fraction. *N Engl J Med* 2019;381(21):1995–2008

20. Zinman B, Wanner C, Lachin JM, et al. Empagliflozin, cardiovascular outcomes, and mortality in type 2 diabetes. *N Engl J Med* 2015;373(22):2117–2128

21. Perkovic V, Jardine MJ, Neal B, et al. Canagliflozin and renal outcomes in type 2 diabetes and nephropathy. *N Engl J Med* 2019;380(24):2295–2306

22. Heerspink HJL, Stefánsson BV, Correa-Rotter R, et al. Dapagliflozin in patients with chronic kidney disease. *N Engl J Med* 2020;383(15):1436–1446

23. White NH, Cleary PA, Dahms W, et al. Beneficial effects of intensive therapy of diabetes during adolescence: outcomes after the conclusion of the Diabetes Control and Complications Trial (DCCT). *J Pediatr* 2001;139(6):804–812

24. Holman RR, Paul SK, Bethel MA, Matthews DR, Neil HA. 10-year follow-up of intensive glucose control in type 2 diabetes. *N Engl J Med* 2008;359(15):1577–1589

25. LeRoith D, Biessels GJ, Braithwaite SS, et al. Treatment of diabetes in older adults: an Endocrine Society Clinical Practice Guideline. *J Clin Endocrinol Metab* 2019;104(5):1520–1574

26. Toschi E, Slyne C, Sifre K, et al. The relationship between CGM-derived metrics, A1C, and risk of hypoglycemia in older adults with type 1 diabetes. *Diabetes Care* 2020;43(10):2349–2354

27. Sargsyan A, Herman MA. Regulation of glucose production in the pathogenesis of type 2 diabetes. *Curr Diab Rep* 2019;19(9):77

28. Bell KJ, Smart CE, Steil GM, et al. Impact of fat, protein, and glycemic index on postprandial glucose control in type 1 diabetes: implications for intensive diabetes management in the continuous glucose monitoring era. *Diabetes Care* 2015;38(6):1008–1015

29. Cryer PE. Hypoglycemia-associated autonomic failure in diabetes. *Am J Physiol Endocrinol Metab* 2001;281(6):E1115–E1121

30. Cryer PE, Davis SN, Shamoon H. Hypoglycemia in diabetes. *Diabetes Care* 2003;26(6):1902–1912

31. Cryer PE. Mechanisms of sympathoadrenal failure and hypoglycemia in diabetes. *J Clin Invest* 2006;116(6):1470–1473

32. Cryer PE. Mechanisms of hypoglycemia-associated autonomic failure in diabetes. *N Engl J Med* 2013;369(4):362–372

The Team Approach

Highlights
The Team Approach

- Multidisciplinary team management is an effective and efficient approach to providing multidimensional care and support for optimal diabetes treatment.
- Multidisciplinary team management provides the patient with
  - medical diagnosis and treatment,
  - focused diabetes self-management education and support and tools for self-management,
  - medical nutrition therapy and nutrition management assistance, and
  - psychosocial evaluation and support.
- Team management necessitates
  - identification of a shared philosophy of care and common treatment goals,
  - collaborative decision-making and mutual respect,
  - open and ongoing communication, and
  - active involvement by all team members.
- The treatment plan must be individualized with the person with diabetes at the center of the care team and incorporate
  - medical priorities and concerns;
  - the patient's abilities, motivation, readiness for self-management; and
  - the patient's social support and access to resources.
- Active teamwork requires the patient to
  - become involved in daily self-care;
  - acquire the skills necessary to make reasoned decisions;
  - implement the necessary treatment interventions;
  - maintain frequent, open, and honest communication with healthcare providers; and
  - advocate for personal self-care needs.

- Healthcare provider responsibilities are to
  - provide time-sensitive intensification of therapies,
  - provide a proactive rather than a reactive care plan,
  - develop rapport and trust through nonjudgmental communication,
  - collaboratively establish treatment goals,
  - inform and educate,
  - negotiate needed lifestyle changes, and
  - facilitate achievement of knowledgeable independence in self-care.
- Effective team communication requires
  - clear role expectations,
  - flexible professional boundaries,
  - shared responsibility,
  - an open approach to management interventions, and
  - mutual respect among team members.
- Patients should hear the same message from team members to avoid confusion and undermining of treatment.

The Team Approach

The American Diabetes Association supports the position that intensive diabetes management should be utilized for most patients with diabetes.[1] Similar to other chronic diseases, diabetes is best managed using a chronic care model.[2] This includes working with the person with diabetes at the center of the care team, formulating sustainable strategies to manage diabetes and its complications, and open communication among all members of the care team.[1] Management of diabetes requires that lifestyle and behavior be addressed in order for medical and nutrition interventions to be accepted and successfully integrated into the daily routine. Team based care is based on diabetes self-management education and support (DSME/S), which is a "process of facilitating the knowledge, skills, and ability necessary for diabetes self-care."[3] For DSME/S to be meaningful, specialized clinical knowledge is provided by a team including nurses, dietitians, pharmacists, and other professionals in addition to the prescribing provider.[4] The ultimate goals of this method of care delivery are to improve clinical outcomes, health status, and quality of life.[5]

Multidisciplinary team management has become the gold standard for providing the multidimensional care and support that diabetes demands.[1,4] This approach emphasizes focused diabetes education, nutrition management, interventions that enhance physical fitness, and psychosocial support, all of which complement the traditional medical model that includes diagnosis and treatment. Lack of time, a fragmented healthcare delivery system, and lack of multidimensional expertise are significant constraints to providing optimal multidisciplinary care. Intensive diabetes management cannot be expected to occur in the context of two to four brief medical management visits per year.[4] In stark contrast, the intensive management group of the Diabetes Control and Complications Trial (DCCT) had monthly appointments with the study healthcare team and even more frequent phone calls from staff who reviewed blood glucose patterns and adjusted insulin regimens.[6,7] Although this level of intervention may not be feasible within the bounds of our current healthcare models, providing multidisciplinary care may be the best available approximation and compromise.

Management of diabetes necessitates active involvement, open communication, and mutual understanding by both the patient and the healthcare team (see Table 2.1). Ongoing diabetes care can be most effectively carried out in the context of this trusting relationship.[8,9]

Table 2.1—Factors That Improve Team Function

- Developing common goals and objectives
- Defining role expectations of each team member, *including* the patient
- Identifying and addressing barriers to care
- Providing evidence-based and structured care
- Offering open communication to solicit feedback in a timely manner

INTEGRATED DIABETES MANAGEMENT TEAM

An integrated diabetes management team is guided in self-care practices and management interventions by the team's professional members. The patient's self-management efforts can be further supported by individuals who play important roles in the patient's day-to-day life, such as spouses, significant others, parents, children, teachers, friends, and coworkers.[10] Within the healthcare system, paraprofessionals including medical assistants, community health workers, peer educators, social workers, and case managers may also play supportive roles.[3,4] With advances in diabetes technology, the care team may also include "connected care" systems, such as continuous glucose monitors, smartphone apps, and automatic coaching devices.[11] The patient must be engaged, however, to make the commitment to self-care and be an active participant in his or her healthcare; otherwise, progress will be limited. Active participation includes

- demonstrating commitment to work at intensive treatment,
- acquiring the necessary skills to manage treatment changes,
- making ongoing decisions regarding daily management,
- identifying and addressing factors affecting the treatment plan, and
- maintaining frequent, open, and honest communication with the healthcare team.

Healthcare providers have the responsibility to inform and educate the patient about available treatment options, work with the patient to establish recommended treatment goals, and foster self-management skills to make needed lifestyle changes (see Table 2.2).[12] The goal of these interventions is to enhance knowledge, facilitate empowerment over one's condition, and promote independent self-care based on the individual's abilities.[10,13,14] This may include customizing a care team and strategies based on the patient's language, literacy, and numeracy skills; cultural and socioeconomic backgrounds; and comorbid conditions.[15] It is known that rates of diabetes and clinical outcomes are influenced by social determinants of health, including but not limited to housing, food security, and social support.[16] It is therefore imperative for the care team to be mindful of the various factors in patients' lives that may impact their diabetes management. Ongoing communication (problem-solving, feedback, and support) should further guide the patient's efforts. Patient education programs should incorporate

- technical skills training,
- guidelines for individualized dietary and physical activity approaches,

Table 2.2—Healthcare Provider Responsibilities

- Utilize open and nonjudgmental communication
- Offer communication in a way that is both efficient and effective, which may include telemedicine or remote-care modalities
- Understand aspects of the patient's life outside of diabetes, especially those that might affect diabetes management
- Know the current American Diabetes Association's Clinical Practice Recommendations and their scientific and clinical basis
- Maintain up to date training in diabetes self-management education
- Implement an effective treatment plan through ongoing patient education and communication
- Foster appropriate independence in self-care practices
- Provide ongoing feedback and support

- problem-solving techniques,
- glucose pattern recognition,
- guidance regarding risk management and management of diabetes comorbidities, and
- identification of interpersonal and practical supports that will enable patients to intensify their care regimen and maintain their progress.

If the healthcare team is not readily available or adequately prepared with the knowledge, skills, and resources necessary to implement intensive diabetes management, or it is not committed to utilization of this form of therapy, it would be better to refer patients wanting this approach to centers that are prepared to undertake this endeavor.[4] Table 2.3 outlines the characteristics of well-functioning healthcare teams. A collaborative relationship between the diabetes team and the primary care provider is also crucial to the success and effectiveness of the patient's treatment plan. This relationship is particularly important because the primary care provider is often the recipient of after-hours calls from patients and may have more contact with the patient compared to the specialty provider.

Table 2.3—Characteristics of a Well-Functioning Healthcare Team

- Belief in the benefits of intensive diabetes management
- Respect for other team members, *including* the patient
- Appreciation for the value of patient–provider collaboration
- Participation in regular and ongoing communication among team members to provide consistent information to patients
- Ability to provide or to access multidisciplinary education and healthcare expertise
- Availability of 24-h assistance for problem-solving

DEFINING TEAM MEMBERS' ROLES

A clear understanding of the team's practice pattern and the responsibilities of individual team members is a key requirement for effective team functioning. Each member's contribution to the team effort should be determined by his or her educational background, credentials, individual abilities, experience, interests, and overall goals of team operation. Importantly, the multidisciplinary team has been described as providing complementary skills, more contact time for the assessment and treatment of patients, and assisting patients with learning diabetes self-care and preventative care through consistent messages, repetition of information, reinforcement and feedback of self-care behaviors, and greater availability to deal with diabetes concerns that may arise.[17,18] Typical roles and responsibilities for the physician, diabetes care and education specialist, dietitian, and mental health professional members of the diabetes care team are listed in Table 2.4.[12,19] Note that these roles have considerable overlap, and few roles are exclusive.

Table 2.4 — Typical Roles and Responsibilities of the Diabetes Care Team Members

- Role of the prescriber
  - Establish medical diagnosis and define treatment plan
  - Provide rationale for treatment
  - Collaborate openly with the patient and team to design and implement a treatment plan
  - Oversee overall patient management
  - Overcome therapeutic inertia
  - Provide patient and family support
- Role of the diabetes care and education specialist
  - Provide self-care assessment
  - Oversee patient education: self-management skills, technical proficiency, and problem-solving
  - Offer family education and assessment
  - Complement physician visits with more frequent contact: acute problem management and blood glucose pattern review
  - Provide patient and family support
- Role of the dietitian
  - Offer nutrition assessment
  - Provide specialized medical nutrition therapy and meal plan development
  - Complement physician visits with more frequent contact: meal plan integration or modification and blood glucose pattern review
  - Provide patient and family support
- Role of mental health professional
  - Elicit and address patient and family concerns and fears about treatment regimen and possible adverse events
  - Identify treatment obstacles
  - Identify sources of support in the patient's daily life
  - Provide patient and family support
  - Offer psychological assessment and treatment or referral as needed

The team's effectiveness will be influenced by the ability of its members to collaborate through mutual respect, a shared philosophy of treatment, consistent goals for patient care, and regular and consistent communication. Within the multidisciplinary framework, no team member operates in isolation. Instead, expertise and strengths are combined to achieve comprehensive, patient-centered care.[20] Multidisciplinary care serves to extend the scope and availability of assessment, intervention, follow-up, and treatment for the individual with diabetes. The care team can also provide additional support in preventative care efforts, which is especially important in diabetes care.[21]

Multidisciplinary diabetes management cannot be limited to those teams working within one department or one institution. Comprehensive team management also can operate in a team composed of members located at different sites. For this approach to be effective, emphasis must be placed on ongoing, accurate, and complete communication among the team members.[22] Regardless of how the team is created, its members must share common treatment goals and cooperate in treatment decisions to minimize confusion and conflict for the patient (see the section Team Communication).

Providers practicing in situations with little access to multidisciplinary care will need to become knowledgeable in all aspects of intensive management to the best of their ability. Nontraditional care teams may also be utilized, in particular in rural settings or in areas with limited access to healthcare. These may include telemedicine visits, shared medical visits, and group education.[23]

TEAM COMMUNICATION

Effective team communication includes an understanding of how to engage with patients and the development of a consistent and unified treatment message and approach (see Table 2.5). Conflicting messages from providers confuse patients and diminish treatment effectiveness.[22]

Within treatment teams, role definitions and boundaries serve to define certain tasks. The complex nature of diabetes management necessitates flexibility in these boundaries, however, resulting in a blending of roles and sharing of responsibilities.

Team meetings provide an opportunity for members to readily communicate with each other and to maintain a focused approach to their healthcare practices

Table 2.5—Fostering Effective Team Communication

- Have a common philosophy and messaging
- Create well-defined expectations
- Be flexible with regard to professional boundaries
- Share responsibility
- Show mutual respect for all team members
- Document clinical updates in a timely manner in the electronic medical record or health record

Table 2.6—Conducting Effective Team Meetings

- Maintain focus on common philosophy, goals, and mutual respect
- Review patient progress or problems
- Identify individual patient behaviors that can be targeted by the team to enhance treatment efficacy
- Identify healthcare system or clinic trends
- Provide active, multidisciplinary problem solving
- Offer support for team members

(see Table 2.6). If held on a regular basis, team meetings facilitate review of individual patient problems or progress, identify healthcare system obstacles and patient care trends, and provide a forum for active problem-solving. Team meetings also facilitate ongoing support among the healthcare providers struggling with particularly difficult patient situations and decrease conflicts within the team. Alternative or adjunctive methods of communication may involve patient rounds or journal clubs. Effective communication can improve cohesion among the team and help develop common approaches to patient care.[12]

CONCLUSION

A multidisciplinary team approach to diabetes treatment is likely the best way to provide patients with a holistic approach to diabetes care—one that addresses the complex parts of day-to-day management. In the present healthcare system, it is difficult for any single clinician to intensively manage diabetes with its many comorbidities and challenging lifestyle recommendations. The team allows for more effective treatment by having a diverse staff that offers complementary skills and more contact time for assessment and treatment of patients, developing treatment relationships, and supporting patients in learning diabetes self-care. Furthermore, as the diabetes epidemic increases, primary care physicians more frequently manage complicated diabetes patients who present with many comorbidities. This increases the number of clinical concerns that need to be addressed during primary care visits and results in less available physician time to address each individual problem. Therefore, team members' increased availability and familiarity with diabetes patients may be crucial to improved diabetes care.

REFERENCES

1. American Diabetes Association. Improving care and promoting health in populations. *Diabetes Care* 2021;44(Suppl. 1):S7–S14

2. Stellefson M, Dipnarine K, Stopka C. The chronic care model and diabetes management in US primary care settings: a systematic review. *Prev Chronic Dis* 2013;10:E26

3. Kelley AT, Nocon RS, O'Brien MJ. Diabetes management in community health centers: a review of policies and programs. *Curr Diab Rep* 2020;20(2):8

4. Powers MA, Bardsley JK, Cypress M, et al. Diabetes self-management education and support in adults with type 2 diabetes: a consensus report of the American Diabetes Association, the Association of Diabetes Care & Education Specialists, the Academy of Nutrition and Dietetics, the American Academy of Family Physicians, the American Academy of PAs, the American Association of Nurse Practitioners, and the American Pharmacists Association. *Diabetes Care* 2020;43(7):1636–1649

5. Powers MA, Bardsley J, Cypress M, et al. Diabetes self-management education and support in type 2 diabetes. *Diabetes Educ* 2017;43(1):40–53

6. Lachin JM, Genuth S, Cleary P, Davis MD, Nathan DM. Retinopathy and nephropathy in patients with type 1 diabetes four years after a trial of intensive therapy. *N Engl J Med* 2000;342(6):381–389

7. Nathan DM, Genuth S, Lachin J, et al. The effect of intensive treatment of diabetes on the development and progression of long-term complications in insulin-dependent diabetes mellitus. *N Engl J Med* 1993;329(14):977–986

8. Tamhane S, Rodriguez-Gutierrez R, Hargraves I, Montori VM. Shared decision-making in diabetes care. *Curr Diab Rep* 2015;15(12):112

9. Schillinger D, Piette J, Grumbach K, et al. Closing the loop: physician communication with diabetic patients who have low health literacy. *Arch Intern Med* 2003;163(1):83–90

10. Rubin R. Facilitating self-care in people with diabetes. *Diabetes Spectr* 2001;14(2):55–57

11. Levine BJ, Close KL, Gabbay RA. Reviewing U.S. connected diabetes care: the newest member of the team. *Diabetes Technol Ther* 2020;22(1):1–9

12. National Diabetes Education Program, National Institutes of Health. *Redesigning the Heath Care Team: Diabetes Prevention and Lifelong Management.* Bethesda, MD, U.S. Department of Health and Human Services, 2011

13. Brink SJ, Miller M, Moltz KC. Education and multidisciplinary team care concepts for pediatric and adolescent diabetes mellitus. *J Pediatr Endocrinol Metab* 2002;15(8):1113–1130

14. Caravalho JY, Saylor CR. An evaluation of a nurse case-managed program for children with diabetes. *Pediatr Nurs* 2000;26(3):296–300

15. Anderson D. Diabetes self-management in a community health center: improving health behaviors and clinical outcomes for underserved patients. *Clin Diabetes* 2008;26(1):22–27

16. Hill-Briggs F, Adler NE, Berkowitz SA, et al. Social determinants of health and diabetes: a scientific review. *Diabetes Care* 2020;44(1):258–279

17. Ritholz MD, Beverly EA, Abrahamson MJ, et al. Physicians' perceptions of the type 2 diabetes multi-disciplinary treatment team: a qualitative study. *Diabetes Educ* 2011;37(6):794–800

18. Wagner EH. The role of patient care teams in chronic disease management. *BMJ* 2000;320(7234):569–572

19. Davidson P, Ross T, Castor C. Academy of Nutrition and Dietetics: revised 2017 standards of practice and standards of professional performance for registered dietitian nutritionists (competent, proficient, and expert) in diabetes care. *J Acad Nutr Diet* 2018;118(5):932–946

20. Glasgow RE, Hiss RG, Anderson RM, et al. Report of the Health Care Delivery Work Group: behavioral research related to the establishment of a chronic disease model for diabetes care. *Diabetes Care* 2001;24(1):124–130

21. Davidson MB. Effect of nurse-directed diabetes care in a minority population. *Diabetes Care* 2003;26(8):2281–2287

22. Lorenz RA, Bubb J, Davis D, et al. Changing behavior: practical lessons from the Diabetes Control and Complications Trial. *Diabetes Care* 1996;19(6):648–652

23. Lee SWH, Chan CKY, Chua SS, Chaiyakunapruk N. Comparative effectiveness of telemedicine strategies on type 2 diabetes management: a systematic review and network meta-analysis. *Sci Rep* 2017;7(1):12680.

Diabetes Self-Management Support and Education

Highlights

Integration of the Team Approach

Diabetes Education

Assessment

Instruction
    Environment
    Planning
    Content
    Sequencing of Diabetes Education
    Education Strategies

Motivation and Support

Action Planning

Evaluation

Documentation

Conclusion

References

Highlights
Diabetes Self-Management
Support and Education

- The patient receiving intensive diabetes management must translate new information and skills into behavior change. Each interaction with the patient is an opportunity for the healthcare provider to teach, reinforce, and encourage. The team approach is best exemplified when information is consistent among team members.

- The patient's readiness to learn new information is a necessary component of any negotiated education plan. The individual will be most receptive when the education is relevant to his or her current needs. In addition, eliciting the patient's commitment to behavior change is another integral component of any education program.

- Education assessment includes information about the patient's knowledge, skills, attitudes, and current diabetes care behaviors. The patient must possess a basic level of understanding before learning the more sophisticated aspects of intensive diabetes management.

- Education is communication and requires careful planning and delivery of pertinent information. Education should be sequenced to build on existing knowledge. Teaching methods include the use of print and audiovisual media. These items must be content-appropriate, readable, and culturally sensitive.

- Intensive diabetes management requires active patient involvement and problem-solving. As part of their education, some individuals may need assistance in actively participating in their care.

- Evaluating the success of patient education can be practical and quick. By using a series of "what-if" questions, the educator is able to assess the patient's problem-solving abilities.

- Documenting and communicating key aspects of the education experience allows diabetes care and education specialists to share information with primary care and referring physicians and other healthcare providers.

Diabetes Self-Management Support and Education

It is well-established that diabetes self-management support (DSMS) and diabetes self-management education and support (DSME/S) are integral to the success of an intensive management program. Patients embarking on the road to improved glycemic control must not only understand the complexities of diabetes and perform the necessary technical skills, but also have confidence in the management strategies and their self-management abilities. Intensive management requires patients to assume an active role in management decisions on a daily basis. To do this safely and effectively, patients need a supportive, knowledgeable, and accessible professional healthcare team. The purpose of DSME/S is to enhance the knowledge, confidence, and self-efficacy of people with diabetes and to support the acceptance of responsibility for their self-management.

DSME/S is successful when patients are able to translate the information and skills into behavior change. Consequently, diabetes education and support is more than a lecture or two on how to control the disease. Instead, it is an ongoing program of assessment, instruction, support, negotiation, and evaluation delivered by a team of diabetes professionals.

INTEGRATION OF THE TEAM APPROACH

A coordinated team of professionals provides depth to the patient's DSME/S. The physician; nurse manager, educator, or clinician; dietitian; the mental health professional; and the pharmacist and exercise physiologist all contribute particular skills and focus. The physician may create a team by referring to a community-based patient education program or to local diabetes care and education specialists. The American Diabetes Association and the Association of Diabetes Care and Education Specialists (ADCES, formally known as AADE) maintain lists of nationally recognized or accredited education programs. In addition, the ADCES assists in locating local diabetes care and education specialists. The National Certification Board for Diabetes Educators has recently transitioned to a new name, The Certification Board for Diabetes Care and Education, and keeps a roster of certified individuals. The well-known credential Certified Diabetes Educator (CDE) has similarly been transitioned to Certified Diabetes Care and Education Specialist (CDCES) in order to more accurately reflect the multifaceted, integral role these individuals play in providing collaborative, person-centered diabetes care.[1]

Diabetes education should never stand alone. Instead, it is a component of the care and management of the patient with diabetes. All members of the treatment team are teachers. Each contact with the patient is an opportunity to teach, reinforce, or evaluate the effect of teaching.

Information must be consistent across professionals. This consistency allows the patient to develop the necessary trust in the management plan and in the healthcare providers. Education materials must be consistent in content. Consequently, each team member should know what the others are teaching.

Diabetes care and education specialists are frequently underutilized even though they represent a cornerstone of diabetes management.[2] DSME/S has clearly established efficacy in improving multiple health outcomes, quality of life, and has proven cost-effectiveness.[1,2] A few of the numerous benefits include lowering of hemoglobin A_{1c} (A1C), reduced emergency department visits and hospital admissions, fewer hypoglycemic events, less diabetes-related distress, and improved self-efficacy and coping mechanisms. In addition, costs are widely reimbursed by multiple insurance plans as long as DSME/S programs meet certification and billing requirements.

DIABETES EDUCATION

Diabetes information should be taught with the understanding that learning about and adjusting to the condition is an ongoing process. One class or a series of classes at diagnosis does not confer lifelong "immunity." Instead, education should be viewed as a treatment that requires periodic boosters and lifelong learning. There are four critical periods where DSME/S should be emphasized: at diagnosis, annually and/or when not meeting treatment targets, when diabetes complications develop, and when transitions in life and care occur.[1]

Patients vary in their willingness or readiness to learn. At times, learner readiness is high, including when new research findings are released, when new medications are available, when complications occur, and when developmental changes arise. At these times, the diabetes care team should capitalize on these "teachable moments" because the patient's motivation and interest are peaking.[3]

Ongoing DSMS also helps people with diabetes maintain effective self-management throughout a lifetime of diabetes as they face new challenges and as treatment advances become available.[4] DSME/S helps patients optimize metabolic control, prevent and manage complications, and maximize quality of life in a cost-effective manner.[4,5]

DSMS and DSME/S are the ongoing processes of facilitating the knowledge, skill, and ability necessary for self-care.[1] This process incorporates the needs, goals, and life experiences of the person with diabetes. The overall objectives of DSMS and DSME/S are to support informed decision-making, self-care behaviors, problem-solving, and active collaboration with the healthcare team to improve clinical outcomes, health status, and quality of life in a cost-effective manner.[6]

ASSESSMENT

The first step in developing an individual education plan is to gather information about the patient's current knowledge, skills, attitudes, behaviors, and environment.[7] Because intensive management is so dependent on the patient's involvement and decision-making, certain basic facts and skills are necessary. Table 3.1 lists the prerequisite information for patients entering an intensive management program. In addition to having this prerequisite information, the patient must accurately and safely perform certain self-management skills. These skills include

- using a blood glucose meter and/or continuous glucose monitoring (CGM) device,
- troubleshooting problems with glucose measurements,
- testing urine or blood ketones,
- record keeping or data management, and
- preparing and delivering insulin.

A careful education assessment includes the following:

- **Personal and socioeconomic information:** age; developmental stage; level of formal education; family composition; significant others; cultural, religious, and ethnic factors; resources; health insurance; and transportation

Table 3.1 — Basic Facts for the Candidate for Intensive Diabetes Management

- Medication: insulin action and insulin regimens
- Rationale for self-monitoring of blood glucose: frequency of checking, goals, patterns
- A1C: monitoring frequency, goals
- Nutrition management
  - Healthy food choices
  - Role of major nutrients: effect on blood glucose levels
  - Carbohydrate counting
  - Sick-day management
  - Label reading
  - Dining out and convenience foods
- Effect of exercise
- Interaction of exercise, nutrition, and medication
- Hypoglycemia: causes, treatment, prevention
- Glucagon
- Identifying the dawn phenomenon
- Hyperglycemia: causes, treatment, prevention
- Ketoacidosis: causes, treatment, prevention
- Complications: causes, symptoms, prevention, monitoring
- Effect of daily living on diabetes control
  - Alcohol consumption
  - Work schedules
  - Traveling
  - Illness or medications and control

Table 3.2—Eliciting the Patient's Beliefs

- What has been your experience with chronic health problems?
- How do you usually deal with success and failure?
- How has your diabetes affected your family?
- What worries or concerns you most about having diabetes?
- How do you typically learn new things?
- What one thing would you tell someone newly diagnosed with diabetes?
- What is the hardest part of diabetes management?
- What do you hope improved diabetes management will do for you?

- **Diabetes information:** type and duration of diabetes, current and previous management approaches, acute and chronic complications, previous diabetes education, and successes as well as challenges with adherence
- **Other medical information:** height, weight, blood pressure, pertinent laboratory values (e.g., blood glucose, A1C, lipids, albumin), other illnesses, other medications, general health status, visual and hearing acuity, and motor skills
- **Lifestyle factors:** use of alcohol, tobacco, or other social drugs; physical activity; stressors; occupation; recreation; and social support systems
- **Nutrition information:** meal and snack times, locations, and typical foods; food preferences and intolerances; previous experience with "diets"; and previous nutrition education
- **Education factors:** learning style, literacy, numeracy, native language, readiness to learn, decision-making skills, health information–seeking behaviors, technology preferences, health beliefs (e.g., locus of control, confidence, experience with other chronic illnesses, coping patterns, fears, concerns), ability and willingness to seek help, expectations of and capacity to deal with failure, assertiveness skills, organizational skills, response to an education plan, and motivators or barriers

Some questions to elicit the patient's beliefs and concerns are listed in Table 3.2.

INSTRUCTION

ENVIRONMENT

The learning environment includes not only the physical facility but also the characteristics of the instructor who facilitates the learning. To help the patient focus on the content, the location should be quiet, with adequate lighting, and free from distractions. Such attention to the environment decreases the cognitive load to efficient learning. Qualities of the teacher that promote learning are listed in Table 3.3.

The educator must draw from an extensive knowledge base while translating this knowledge into language understandable to the patient-learner. Furthermore, the

Table 3.3—Qualities and Competencies of the Teacher

- Possesses a knowledge base that is current and extensive
- Holds a personal belief that patients can learn
- Is empathetic
- Is nonjudgmental
- Is adaptable: flexible in using a variety of teaching approaches
- Is able to
  - Individualize information
  - Encourage questions
  - Allow adequate time for patients to answer
  - Use clear, simple, concrete explanations
  - Sequence educational topics
  - Involve others as needed
  - Repeat and reinforce facts
  - Provide for reflection and review of content
  - Evaluate understanding
  - Provide focused and timely feedback

educator must be able to adjust an educational agenda to meet the learner's needs. For example, the educator may have determined that the patient should hear about different insulin programs, whereas the patient may want to learn about counting carbohydrates. Adult learners always will focus on what the education encounter will mean to them. The educator is most successful when able to adapt to changes in the teaching agenda.

Education is a process of communication and reception of information. Throughout the education session, the educator assesses the learner's understanding. By asking the patient to restate the information or to use the information to solve a problem, the educator is then able to evaluate learning.

PLANNING

As the assessment proceeds, the educator will identify topics and teaching approaches that are most appropriate for the patient. Shared goal setting is important. The plan for the education program becomes a negotiation between the teacher and learner.[7]

Often, the patient doesn't know what he or she needs to know and may be resistant to new information. The educator's job is to gently challenge the patient's knowledge while presenting new information. The educator may need to remind the patient that medical knowledge about diabetes changes rapidly and old information is being replaced with new ways of handling the disease.

The educator's job is to engage the patient-learner in the education by listening to the learner's needs and building trust. The patient is more likely to remain interested when the content is meaningful and consistent with what the patient already knows. Strategies to maintain interest include using interactive teaching approaches and incorporating time for review and reflection of new content.[8,9]

CONTENT

Topics especially pertinent for the patient implementing intensive diabetes management include

- nutrition guidelines and the effect of food on glycemic control,
- medication action and dosage adjustment,
- impact of exercise on blood glucose control,
- monitoring,
- prevention and detection of chronic complications,
- the role of diabetes technology in intensive management
- behavior change strategies, and
- problem-solving.

A comprehensive curriculum list is included in Table 3.4.

SEQUENCING OF DIABETES EDUCATION

There is far too much information on intensive management to deliver in one session. Effective diabetes education occurs over several contacts with the patient.[10] The most meaningful education sessions build on the patient's existing knowledge and on content from previous sessions. For instance, one session may be devoted to a discussion about insulin regimens, the interpretation of blood glucose results, and recordkeeping. The next session may focus on problem-solving by reviewing blood glucose records and discussing and demonstrating insulin adjustment techniques.

EDUCATION STRATEGIES

Adults learn best when the information is immediately useful and relevant. Thus, teaching a patient to implement an intensive management plan must include enough time to practice the decision-making required and focus on information needed to implement the treatment plan. For example, if the patient will be using an algorithm to adjust insulin doses, then the educator must plan for opportunities to practice using that algorithm.

The educator should have a repertoire of real-life examples to use when teaching. Most individuals need help to develop the judgment and problem-solving needed to make diabetes decisions. Consider, for instance, what a patient must evaluate in choosing an insulin dose before a meal. How much carbohydrate and fat will be consumed? What is the current blood glucose level? How far from target is the blood glucose level? What range of insulin doses tends to work for this mealtime? What will the exercise level be in the next several hours? How long should the time between injection and meal be? Working through several examples with the patient allows the educator to model good decision-making. Decision-making and problem-solving skills are acquired and improved through practice. Mistakes are part of the learning process. The educator must create opportunities for practice and an environment in which errors and misjudgments are used to learn, not criticize.

Table 3.4—Curriculum for Intensive Management

- Diabetes overview and review
  - DCCT results: long-term control and benefits
  - Benefits, risks, and management options for improving glucose control
- Stress and psychosocial adjustment
  - Effect of stress on control
  - Identifying stressors
  - Anticipating stress
  - Problem-solving: stress management techniques
- Family involvement and social support
  - Sharing diabetes care: when and how
  - Seeking help
  - Joining support groups
  - Doing volunteer work
- Nutrition
  - Role of nutrients
  - Glycemic impact
  - Label reading
  - Advanced carbohydrate counting or other meal-planning approaches
  - Alcohol: effect and use
  - Dining out versus cooking in (adapting recipes)
  - Problem-solving: evaluating the effect of food adjustments and changes
- Exercise and activity
  - Effect of exercise
  - Exercise physiology
  - Prolonged effect, late post-exercise hypoglycemia
  - Planning pre-exercise food or insulin
  - Problem-solving: evaluating effect of exercise
- Diabetes medication
  - Insulin and other noninsulin injectable medications: storage, preparation, site selection, injection
  - Medication injection delivery systems: technical training for use of pens and pumps
  - Problem-solving: insulin dose changes
    - Using results of monitoring to evaluate blood glucose patterns and variability
    - Basal changes
    - Bolus changes (i.e., algorithms)
    - Supplemental doses or sensitivity (correction) factors
    - Evaluating and verifying the effect of dose adjustment
    - When to call the diabetes team
- Monitoring
  - Blood glucose meter use: technique, meter care, troubleshooting
  - Fingerstick or alternative site technique, care of skin
  - Continuous glucose monitoring
  - Record keeping and data management
  - Understanding and using glucose results
  - When to check urine or blood ketones, and interpretation of results
  - Relationship among nutrition, exercise, medication, and blood glucose levels
  - Effect of unusual days on glucose control
    - Travel
    - Varying work schedules
  - Anticipating changes and making adjustments

DCCT, Diabetes Control and Complications Trial.

Table 3.4—Curriculum for Intensive Management (*Continued*)

- Prevention, detection, and treatment of acute complications
  - Identifying symptoms and causes of hypoglycemia
  - Understanding how symptoms may change as glycemic control improves
  - Glucagon: when to use, who to train, precautions
  - Symptoms and causes of hyperglycemia and its management
  - Diabetic ketoacidosis
- Prevention, detection, and treatment of chronic complications
  - Detection of problems: routine health follow-up and diabetes-specific follow-up
  - Effect of intensification on existing complications
  - Foot, skin, and dental care
    - Injection sites
    - Prevention of infections
    - Dental prophylaxis
- Behavior change strategies, goal setting, negotiation skills, and problem-solving
  - Decision-making skills
  - Problem-solving approaches
  - Interacting with the diabetes team
- Preconception, pregnancy, and postpartum management
- Use of healthcare systems and community resources
  - Creating a diabetes management team
  - Financial impact and cost-saving strategies for intensive diabetes management

Other approaches include using print, audiovisual, and web-based materials. Many excellent materials are available from manufacturers of diabetes supplies. These materials, however, must be evaluated individually for appropriate content, readability, and cultural sensitivity. Interactive educational materials—for example, computer programs, food models, self-instructional materials, and games—add variety to the education program and enhance learner engagement in the process.[10] A sample patient education handout is provided in Table 3.5.

Regardless of the methodology for instruction, one of the most effective approaches to encouraging adherence is simple: Provide the literate patient with clear, written instructions. Patients generally remember very little from their time with the clinician or educator. Written instructions can be the educator's most practical tool.

MOTIVATION AND SUPPORT

The process of patient education is intimately connected to behavior change. The educator should assess how the patient will use or transfer the information to action. Simply asking the patient, "How will you try this at home?" or "What things will be easy or hard to do?" often will alert the educator to potential difficulties in adherence. Some questions to elicit the patient's commitment to behavior change are listed in Table 3.6.

Table 3.5—Sample Worksheet for Intensive Diabetes Management in Type 1 Diabetes

Goals for Intensive Blood Glucose Control

	American Diabetes Association guidelines	Personal goals
Preprandial plasma glucose	80–130 mg/dL (4.4–7.2 mmol/L)	____ to ____
Peak postprandial glucose	<180 mg/dL (<10.0 mmol/L) 2 h after the start of a meal	Below ____
A1C	<7%	

Basal Insulin

Time	Type	Dose

Bolus Insulin

Time	Type	Dose	Carbohydrate amount

Carbohydrate-to-Insulin Ratio: Breakfast: ____; Lunch ____; Dinner ____; Bedtime: ____

Correction Insulin Dose: _____ units for every _____ mg/dL blood glucose

ACTION PLANNING

Some patients have adequate diabetes knowledge and wish to participate in their care, but they lack the assertive communication or negotiation skills needed. They may feel intimidated by the healthcare professional or by the system. Yet, patient involvement in treatment decisions is important for the individual on an intensive

Table 3.6—Verifying the Patient's Commitment

- How effective do you think this task will be for you?
- What part of the plan may be hard for you?
- Are you concerned about the time or expense?
- How will you know if the plan is working?
- How certain are you that you can do this?
- What makes you certain or uncertain?
- If now is not the right time for you to begin, when will the time be right?

management program. Because the patient will direct so much of the daily management, his or her commitment to the plan is essential.

The educator may assess commitment and confidence with a simple rating tool. After developing an action plan with the patient, the educator asks the patient to rate how confident he or she feels in following the plan. The patient then rates confidence on a scale of 1 to 10 (1 being not at all confident; 10 being highly confident). The educator then should explore what supports the chosen rating and what is preventing a higher rating. Such exploration reveals motivators or supports as well as barriers to behavior change.

The educator may find that the patient actually needs assistance in communicating his or her needs to the physician. The patient's education plan may include tips on how to participate actively in the treatment plan.

EVALUATION

In a busy practice, patient education often amounts to nothing more than the professional relaying information, with little time directed at assessing how the information is received and implemented. Whether provided in the physician's office or in a formal classroom education setting, evaluating the success of patient education can be quick and easy.

Tests and quizzes have a place in some education programs. The adult learner, however, will remember information that is immediately useful. Education sessions should include sufficient time for reflection on the material discussed. Questions to promote reflection and review are listed in Table 3.7. Using a series of "what-if" questions allows the educator not only to assess level of knowledge but also to determine problem-solving abilities. A sample of such questions is provided in Table 3.8.

Table 3.7—Providing Reflection and Review of Educational Content

- What are the three most important points?
- What questions do you still have?
- What did you find most interesting?
- What did you find most difficult?
- How would you summarize this content?
- How could you learn more about this topic?
- What did you learn that was new to you?
- What do you want always to remember?
- How does this content relate to something you already know?
- What will help you remember this material?
- What did you find most surprising?
- What will be the hardest thing to remember?
- How will you use what you learned today?
- What content will make the most difference for you?

Table 3.8—Evaluating Learning and Problem-Solving

- What would you do if
  - You gave yourself insulin and your restaurant meal was late?
  - You were supposed to take rapid-acting insulin before a meal, but your blood glucose level was 40 mg/dL?
  - You were planning to exercise 1 h after lunch?
  - You awakened with nausea and did not feel like eating?
  - Your blood glucose results did not coincide with how you felt?
- How will you adjust your management plan for special occasions and parties?

DOCUMENTATION

The diabetes care and education specialist is obligated to completely document the education process from assessment through evaluation. Checklists and documentation forms may be created to assist the educator in this task. Sample forms are provided in the section titled Education Recognition Program at https://professional.diabetes.org/diabetes-education. To provide continuity and consistency and to facilitate the team approach, the educator, in addition to documenting the medical record, also should provide follow-up information to the referring physician or prescriber.

CONCLUSION

Patient education and support is integral to the success of intensifying the individual's diabetes management. The patient must be skilled, knowledgeable, and willing to participate fully and successfully in the decisions about daily self-care. The physician, diabetes care and education specialist, and other professionals must form a unified patient care team to ensure that the patient receives consistent and accurate information. Success in providing DSMS and DSMS/E requires attention to patient assessment, individual instruction, and evaluation of patient response and the patient's willingness to participate in their care.

REFERENCES

1. Powers MA, Bardsley JK, Cypress M, Funnell MM, Harms D, Hess-Fischl A, et al. Diabetes self-management education and support in adults with type 2 diabetes: a consensus report of the American Diabetes Association, the Association of Diabetes Care and Education Specialists, the Academy of Nutrition and Dietetics, the American Academy of Family Physicians, the American Academy of PAs, the American Association of Nurse Practitioners, and the American Pharmacists Association. *Diabetes Care* 2020;43(7): 1636–1649

2. Rinker J, Dickinson JK, Litchman ML, Williams AS, Kolb LE, Cox C, Lipman RD. The 2017 Diabetes Educator and the Diabetes Self-Management Education National Practice Survey. *Diabetes Educ* 2018;44(3):260–268

3. Beck J, Greenwood DA, Blanton L, Bollinger ST, Butcher MK, Condon JE, et al. 2017 National Standards for Diabetes Self-Management Education and Support. *Diabetes Care* 2017;40(10):1409–1419

4. Boren SA, Fitzner KA, Panhalkar PS, Specker JE. Costs and benefits associated with diabetes education: a review of the literature. *Diabetes Educ* 2009;35(1):72–96

5. Duncan I, Ahmed T, Li QE, Stetson B, Ruggiero L, Burton K, et al. Assessing the value of the diabetes educator. *Diabetes Educ* 2011;37(5):638–657

6. Mensing C. Comparing the processes: accreditation and recognition. *Diabetes Educ* 2010;36(2):219–243

7. Burke SD, Sherr D, Lipman RD. Partnering with diabetes educators to improve patient outcomes. *Diabetes Metab Syndr Obes* 2014;7:45–53

8. Ehrmann D, Kulzer B, Schipfer M, Lippmann-Grob B, Haak T, Hermanns N. Efficacy of an education program for people with diabetes and insulin pump treatment (INPUT): results from a randomized controlled trial. *Diabetes Care* 2018;41(12):2453–2462

9. Heller SR, Gianfrancesco C, Taylor C, Elliott J. What are the characteristics of the best type 1 diabetes patient education programmes (from diagnosis to long-term care), do they improve outcomes and what is required to make them more effective? *Diabet Med* 2020;37(4):545–554

10. Bodenheimer T. Helping patients improve their health-related behaviors: what system changes do we need? *Dis Manag* 2005;8(5):319–330

Psychosocial Issues

Highlights
Psychosocial Issues

- Active patient engagement with self-care behaviors and the willingness to collaborate on treatment decisions are good indicators of future success with an intensive diabetes management plan. Patient engagement is promoted by an effective patient–clinician relationship and communication. From the outset of treatment, clinicians need to foster patients' active inquiry and participation so that self-care behaviors can be discussed, monitored for mastery and effectiveness, and modified in an ongoing fashion.

- Understanding and addressing the psychosocial factors that may promote or interfere with patients' active engagement in intensive diabetes management is of critical importance. Therefore, psychosocial assessments are beneficial, both before intensification of diabetes management begins and throughout the course of treatment. Diabetes burnout, diabetes distress, depression, anxiety, eating disorders, and substance abuse may interfere with patients' intensive diabetes management and need to be assessed and monitored when patients display difficulties with their intensive management. Thus, the clinician can have increased understanding of the possible reasons for the patients' behavior and, with the assistance of the multidisciplinary treatment team, can begin an effective treatment.

- Clinicians should be aware that depression, diabetes distress, and eating disorders are prevalent in patients with diabetes. As a way to address these psychosocial concerns, clinicians should consider using diabetes-specific screening surveys for diabetes distress or non–diabetes-specific surveys for depression. If screening identifies existing problems, further evaluation by a qualified mental health professional is indicated. The mental health professional may use cognitive-behavioral, interpersonal, or family counseling approaches to assist patients with psychosocial difficulties. In addition, the mental health professional must be included as a member of the multidisciplinary treatment team, which is critically important when engaging the patient with psychosocial difficulties in intensive diabetes treatment.

- Periods of psychological distress are expected in the life course of diabetes. For example, how patients perceive and manage the specter or onset of diabetes complications is important to assess. Patients' negative emotional responses and attitudes toward complications may result in their loss of desire for intensive management. These responses may interact with treatment goals and affect intensive management. Importantly, clinicians need to recognize that these reactions are expected and normative, and patients need support in adapting to their actual or perceived limitations. Furthermore, negative responses should be monitored and addressed, especially if they are continuing for too long a period of time.

■ Patients are more likely to succeed with self-care regimens that are responsive to their lifestyle needs and do not present an overwhelming burden. Therefore, patients should be encouraged to set treatment goals that can best fit their personal lifestyle. These goals should be collaboratively determined by patient and clinician and thereby should be achievable by the patient. Ensure that patients begin intensive treatment by feeling they can meet their goals rather than by setting goals that are too difficult to accomplish, which may lead to self-blame, discouragement, and a sense of failure. Furthermore, periodic lapses in self-care behaviors should be accepted as an expected part of intensive diabetes management. Patients may become tired of the demands of intensive diabetes management, resulting in burnout. Therefore, ongoing monitoring and support from healthcare professionals are essential to the achievement and maintenance of treatment goals.

Psychosocial Issues

Intensive diabetes management has become the gold standard treatment for most patients with type 1 diabetes (T1D) and for many with type 2 diabetes (T2D) who use insulin. It is clear that patients can and will follow a medical regimen that is complex and multifaceted when provided with extensive education and professional support.[1] The Look AHEAD study also showed that when multidisciplinary services are available, user friendly, and personalized, a high degree of adherence with a complex lifestyle-based regimen could be achieved and sustained, and intensive treatment goals for T2D could be met, without detrimental effects to the patient's quality of life.[2]

Consequently, healthcare professionals need to spend time presenting a background of the benefits and barriers for intensive treatment. Clinicians can promote patients' increased understanding of the importance of active involvement with self-care behaviors and collaboration in treatment decisions, which are good indicators of future success with an intensive management plan.[3]

Most importantly, patients' active engagement is necessary for successful diabetes management. To promote this engagement, glucose targets and treatment goals should include and reflect the patient's needs, preferences, and values. Furthermore, understanding and addressing the psychosocial factors that may promote or interfere with patients' active engagement in intensive diabetes management is of critical importance. Thus, psychosocial assessments are beneficial, both before intensive diabetes management begins and throughout the course of treatment. Moreover, active patient engagement requires an effective patient–clinician relationship and open communication to support intensive diabetes management.

PSYCHOLOGICAL FACTORS

Psychological distress or well-being can affect a patient's ability to carry out the behavior and communication necessary to implement and maintain intensive diabetes management. Evaluation of current and prior psychological status by a mental health professional familiar with diabetes should ideally be included with the assessment of the patient's physical status. These evaluations should be an integral and ongoing part of intensive diabetes management. The easiest and most direct methods involve short, standardized screening surveys that can identify psychological factors that might interfere with patient's optimal engagement in intensive diabetes management. Some examples of surveys for diabetes distress include Problem Areas in Diabetes (PAID) and the Diabetes Distress Scale (DDS).[4,5] Some widely used, although not diabetes-specific, surveys for depression include the Patient Health Questionnaire 9 (PHQ-9) and the Center for Epidemiological Studies Depression Scale (CES-D).[6] If screening identifies problems, further evaluation by a qualified mental health professional is indicated. This professional can help with treatment decisions and assist family members and others (such as teachers, friends, or coworkers) to support needed behaviors and attitude changes.

A potential contraindication to intensification is a prior or current diagnosis of a psychiatric illness that impairs an individual's ability to carry out activities of daily living (including diabetes self-care tasks). In addition, clinicians also should consider assessing whether the patient can

- make, evaluate, or implement treatment decisions;
- use appropriate problem-solving skills; and
- maintain close contact with a clinician.

If the patient is found to have deficits in the any of these areas, then appropriate psychosocial supports, such as a mental health professional to provide counseling or a case manager to monitor adverse treatment outcomes (e.g., repeated episodes of diabetic ketoacidosis [DKA]) should be put in place.

Diabetes Burnout

Intensive management places greater burdens on the patient than conventional treatment approaches and therefore may contribute to the potential for diabetes burnout, diabetes distress, depression, and reduced quality of life. The occurrence of complications that produce functional limitations, such as worsening eyesight or decreased mobility resulting from micro- and macrovascular disease, also can be sources of diabetes burnout. Therefore, it is important that clinicians assess patients for burnout through the course of treatment. Some important ways to address diabetes burnout include referral to a mental health professional, meeting with other diabetes patients in support groups, and including the patient's family to help them understand what the patient is feeling and how they can support him or her.

Diabetes Distress and Depression

Studies have shown that many patients with diabetes who display high levels of depressive symptoms also experience high levels of emotional distress stemming from concerns and worries associated with their diabetes and its management.[7] Emotional distress is a single, continuous dimension that includes both content (diabetes and its management and other life stresses) and severity, both of which can be addressed directly in clinical care.[8]

The relationship between depression and diabetes appears to be bidirectional; that is, each may contribute to the other. Depression in individuals with diabetes has been implicated in nonadherence with self-care behaviors, lack of motivation to intensify treatment, reduced quality of life, and worsened glycemia.[9] Depression is underdiagnosed in the diabetes population, and importantly, the American Diabetes Association recommends that older adults (>65 years of age) with diabetes should be considered a high-priority population for depression screening and treatment.[10] When assessing patients, healthcare professionals need to be alert to the following situations, which may contribute to patients' distress or depression:

- Diagnosis of diabetes
- Adverse effects of treatment (e.g., severe hypoglycemia, weight gain, or perceived treatment failure)
- Onset of complications
- Negative effect of diabetes care on lifestyle
- Lack of real or perceived support in the home, work, school, or other social environment
- Change in real or perceived self-image or functional abilities
- Fluctuations in physical well-being and mood associated with changes in glucose levels
- Increased burden, including finances, of medical care

Anxiety

Increased anxiety in people with diabetes can occur at diabetes diagnosis, key life transitions (going to college, getting married, starting first job, pregnancy), and the onset of complications.[11] Fear of hypoglycemia is the most common severe anxiety for people with diabetes, which can lead patients to maintain blood glucose levels above recommended targets, increasing their risk for diabetes complications.[12] Some people with diabetes and depression also have comorbid anxiety disorders, such as generalized anxiety disorder, panic disorder, or posttraumatic stress disorder.[9] Anxiety disorders also can occur without comorbid depression in people with diabetes. Anxiety disorders may complicate diabetes management in the following ways: *1*) distinguishing between feelings of anxiety and symptoms of hypoglycemia may make it difficult to know how and when to respond appropriately to distressing feelings, and *2*) preexisting anxiety may lead to severe anxiety or panic disorders after a person is diagnosed with diabetes and needs to begin using injections or have blood draws.

Fear of hypoglycemia. Individuals vary significantly regarding their risk for hypoglycemia, their ability to recognize hypoglycemia symptoms, and their adaptive behaviors for coping with hypoglycemia, as well as the social support they receive for monitoring, recognizing, and treating episodes of hypoglycemia. Furthermore, the overlap between symptoms of hypoglycemia and anxiety can make recognition of episodes difficult.[12] Some patients may develop a maladaptive fear of hypoglycemia that leads them to actively avoid target glucose levels, which is counterproductive to intensive management. Although training patients, families, and others to recognize and treat hypoglycemia or severe hypoglycemia in their home or work environment is usually part of basic diabetes education, this issue should be revisited whenever diabetes management is intensified.

Patients learn to fear hypoglycemia not only for the potential adverse physical outcomes but also for the lack of control that results from neuroglycopenia. Patients experiencing hypoglycemia may act silly, risqué, angry, or irresponsible; take risks; or withdraw. Altered personality characteristics are common. Low blood glucose levels can affect interactions with partners and coworkers, cause errors in mental processing, or alter physical functioning (e.g., cause automobile accidents), all of which are beyond the control of the patient during a hypoglycemic episode.

Fear of hypoglycemia should be periodically assessed, especially if patients' hemoglobin A_{1c} (A1C) is above target levels. When questioned, a patient may describe inappropriately eliminating or excessively reducing insulin doses in relation to the perceived risk of hypoglycemia. In this situation, patients may *1*) fear an abrupt drop in blood glucose level even if their blood glucose is well above 70 mg/dL, *2*) misinterpret feelings of anxiety as hypoglycemia and inappropriately treat the hypoglycemia without addressing the anxiety, *3*) develop heightened fear following an episode of severe hypoglycemia or after repeated episodes of hypoglycemia, or *4*) aim for a relatively high blood glucose range, above which they feel safer from the risk of hypoglycemia.

Some suggested options for addressing fear of hypoglycemia include the following: *1*) use continuous subcutaneous insulin pump therapy, automated insulin delivery systems, or stand-alone continuous glucose monitoring (CGM); *2*) teach strategies to increase recognition of symptoms; *3*) prevent low blood glucose by proactively temporarily reducing insulin doses; and *4*) increase the frequency of blood glucose monitoring (e.g., before and after exercise, before driving).[13] Modern CGM systems can have a major positive influence on many of the concerns with hypoglycemia, including positive collaborative improvements in marital relationships.[13-15] If fear of hypoglycemia becomes an impediment to achieving optimal glycemia, inclusion of a mental health professional who specializes in diabetes should be considered. Behavioral techniques such as exposure in cases in which patients learn to tolerate lower blood glucose levels in the presence of a therapist or family member are effective strategies.

Needle phobia. Many individuals who must use insulin initially express fear of taking injections but quickly accommodate, out of necessity, to injecting insulin. In most cases, firm expectations for the patient's behavior (along with social support and skill building) effectively reduce fear and anxiety. When anxiety and avoidant behaviors increase around giving injections, needle phobia may be the underlying cause. Avoidant behaviors can include, but are not limited to, rituals that prolong the period before the injection is given, intense expressions of distress (moaning, crying, yelling) accompanied by physical withdrawal from the needle, or frank refusal to take injections.

When needle phobia is suspected, an evaluation by a qualified mental health professional is indicated. Cognitive-behavioral therapy, relaxation techniques, and pharmacotherapy are effective in reducing phobic behavior. Insulin pump therapy also can be considered, although pump malfunctions will still require the use of occasional injections, and insertion of the infusion set may be feared. Inhaled Technosphere mealtime insulin and an injection port (Iport, Medtronic) are other options that may have some value in certain individuals. Regardless of the intervention strategies used, it is important that the patient receive pragmatic and nonjudgmental messages about the necessity of overcoming these fears. At the same time, healthcare professionals need to acknowledge the degree of distress the patient is experiencing so that appropriate psychological treatment can occur.

It is important to include significant others in the behavioral intervention because the patient's anxious behaviors may be inadvertently supported, encouraged, and maintained within the context of family dynamics. A prime example of this is a parent who grimaces and cries every time the child with diabetes receives an injection. The child learns to associate negative emotions and distress with receiving an injection even though he or she may experience little physical pain. In these circumstances, needle phobia may evolve. Thus, the child attempts to avoid a "feared stimulus" and also receives parental support for the avoidant behavior. Therefore, both parent and child would benefit from the behavioral intervention.

Psychological insulin resistance. Psychological insulin resistance is sometimes seen when patients with T2D must begin using insulin.[16] This reaction to beginning insulin may include needle phobia, unreasonable personal beliefs about the meaning of insulin therapy, poor self-efficacy, and a lack of accurate information. Patients also may perceive that starting insulin means that she or he has "failed" diabetes management.[17] Importantly, clinicians need to avoid using the start of insulin as a threat to motivate patients to improve their self-care, because this message implies blame for failure in self-management behavior if and when insulin becomes part of treatment.[17,18] Suggestions for addressing the start of insulin include helping the patient understand the progressive natural course of diabetes; demonstrating how oral medication may not be working anymore, without any fault of the patient; and discussing insulin injections as a powerful and necessary tool to achieve glycemic targets.

Eating Disorders

Type 1 diabetes and eating disorders. Studies suggest an increased risk of eating disorders among female patients with T1D. Intermittent insulin restriction for weight loss purposes has been found to be a common practice among women with T1D.[19] For example, in women and girls with T1D between the ages of 13 and 60 years, 31% reported intentional insulin restriction.[20] Rates of restriction peaked in late adolescence and early adulthood, with 40% of women and girls between the ages of 15 and 30 years reporting intentional restriction.

Even at a subclinical level of severity, restricting insulin places women at heightened risk for the medical complications of diabetes. Women reporting intentional insulin restriction had higher A1C levels (by as much as 2 or more points), more frequent hospital and emergency department visits, more frequent episodes of DKA, and higher rates of neuropathy and retinopathy than women who did not report insulin restriction.[21] Insulin restriction was found to triple the risk of mortality during an 11-year follow-up study. Most important, women who stopped insulin restriction reported thinking differently about insulin and weight, no longer fearing that healthy glycemia and appropriate insulin treatment would automatically lead to weight gain.[22]

Although the large majority of research on eating disorders and T1D focuses on insulin restriction as a central symptom, not all patients with eating disorders and T1D restrict insulin. For example, patients with anorexia and T1D require significantly less insulin by virtue of severe calorie restriction and related weight loss. Their eating disorder may go undetected for a while because their glucose values are likely to be in or below the target range. It may not be until they reach a notably low weight or develop a pattern of recurrent hypoglycemia that their eating disorder is discovered. In addition, patients with bulimia and T1D may not always use insulin restriction to purge calories. For example, they may self-induce vomiting or turn to excessive exercise and other means of purging. These behaviors may not have as strong an impact on glycemia as insulin restriction—possibly making eating disorder detection more difficult in these patients as well.

Clinicians may find it helpful to use screening tools to identify patients with eating disorders or those at risk. The Diabetes Eating Problem Survey–Revised (DEPS-R) is a 16-item self-report questionnaire that takes <10 min to complete.[23] The five-item mSCOFF questionnaire has been adapted to help identify insulin restriction and eating disorder behavior.[24]

Type 2 diabetes and binge eating. Because obesity is a significant risk factor in T2D, recurrent binge eating may increase the chances of developing this form of diabetes. Research indicates that a distinct subgroup of obese adults (20–46%) engage in recurrent binge eating.[25]

The literature on binge eating in T2D has grown in recent years. 14% of the patients with newly diagnosed T2D experienced problems with binge eating, compared with 4% of the age-, sex-, and weight-matched control subjects. Participants in the Look AHEAD study who stopped binge eating were found to be able to lose similar amounts of weight when compared with those who did not report binge eating.[2] Participants with binge eating disorder were younger than participants without eating disorders and reported that their weight problems began at younger ages.[26] These data raise the possibility that recurrent binge eating is a risk factor for developing T2D earlier in life. In fact, in the TODAY Study, which evaluated treatments for T2D in adolescence, participants who reported problems with binge eating had higher rates of extreme obesity.[27]

Treatment recommendations. The International Conference on Eating Disorders and Diabetes Mellitus Guidelines recommend a multidisciplinary team approach, including an endocrinologist or diabetologist, nurse educator, nutritionist with eating disorder or diabetes training, and psychologist or social worker with eating disorder expertise to provide weekly individual therapy. Depending on the level of comorbid depression and anxiety, a psychiatrist may be needed for psychopharmacological evaluation and treatment. Treatment outcome research in eating disorders in the general population supports using cognitive-behavioral therapy in combination with antidepressant medications as the most effective treatment. These approaches need to be adapted to directly address the role of insulin restriction for those patients with this symptom.[28]

Once established as a longstanding behavior pattern, the problem of frequent insulin restriction may be particularly difficult to treat. For this reason, early detection and intervention appear to be crucial. Disordered eating behaviors often are associated with intense shame and secrecy, and thus identifying disordered eating as a common struggle in T1D can help the patient with feelings of isolation and also to decrease shame. As for all patients, build a close patient–clinician relationship characterized by open communication and a nonjudgmental stance. This may make it more likely for the patient to feel comfortable disclosing the problem and turning to the diabetes treatment team for help.

With active insulin restriction, the treatment team must be willing to set incremental goals that the patient feels ready to achieve. The first goal is to establish medical safety by focusing on the prevention of DKA and the acute onset of complications such as painful peripheral neuropathy or vision compromise. Gradually, the team can build toward increased doses of insulin, increases in food intake, greater flexibility in meal plans, regularity of eating routines, more frequent blood glucose monitoring, and the final goal of intensive diabetes management.

Substance Abuse

Alcohol consumption is inversely associated with glycemic targets among diabetes patients and is a marker for poorer adherence to diabetes self-care behaviors.[29] In a study of adolescents with chronic illnesses including T1D, it was found that alcohol and marijuana use are prevalent among youth with chronic medical conditions and that alcohol use was associated with youth who reported regularly forgetting to take their medications.[30] Thus, both before beginning intensive diabetes management and during the course of treatment, it is important for healthcare providers to inquire and educate adolescent and adult patients about alcohol use and the ways that it may interfere with diabetes self-care and impede attainment of optimal glycemia.

Stress

Stressors—positive and negative, long or short term—affect the individual's ability to maintain optimal glycemia. The patient's response to stress should be assessed before intensive treatment is begun to identify regimen strategies that will best maximize individual methods of coping with stress. The identification of stress-related events and symptoms is important in identifying potential causes of high or fluctuating blood glucose levels. One possible impact of stress on diabetes management relates to its way of disrupting daily routines and sometimes realigning priorities for a time. These changes not only influence blood glucose levels, but the physiological impact of stress *per se* may have an effect on glycemia. Furthermore, transient stress causes a state of relative insulin resistance as a result of increased concentrations of counterregulatory hormones and leads to hyperglycemia.[31] The effects of chronic stress on glycemia are not well understood.

Healthcare professionals can help patients evaluate the effects of stressful life events through the use of careful blood glucose monitoring records in which the patient is encouraged to record life events as well as blood glucose levels and insulin doses. The patient can learn how to distinguish symptoms caused by life stress, which in turn may affect blood glucose levels, from symptoms that might be expected from more normative changes in blood glucose levels (e.g., feelings of hunger and light-headedness before a planned meal). Patients practicing intensive management should be encouraged to check blood glucose whenever they feel symptoms or experience psychosocial stress to identify their own pattern of glycemic response. With use of CGM, this is easier to do because of frequency of glucose readings and the ability to identify patterns.

Although stressful lifestyles do not preclude an intensive diabetes management regimen, a patient must learn to cope effectively with changes in blood glucose levels caused by stress and to develop and practice coping behaviors. Intervention strategies for stress reduction can include relaxation techniques, regular exercise regimens, support people or groups, medications, and changes in the diabetes management regimen. Intervention strategies should be tailored to the source of the stress, the patient's glycemic response, and the resources (psychological and other) the patient possesses to cope with the stressor.[32]

Patterns of eating in response to stress also need to be addressed for individuals with both T1D and T2D. Patients need counseling to develop coping skills for maintaining glucose levels within the acceptable range through exercise, insulin, or medication modifications when stress-related or emotional eating is identified. Identification of stressors that impede maintenance of optimal glycemia and the development of coping strategies may best be achieved with the help of a mental health professional familiar with diabetes who is integrated into the diabetes care team.

Diabetes Complications

Informing patients about the relationship between intensive treatment and lessening complications may help motivate patients' active participation. Patients sometimes develop negative attitudes about the inevitable development of complications, which may occur when attempts to achieve desired glycemic targets have not succeeded. Success with short-term goals can help alter patient attitudes about the inevitability of complications and may bolster intentions to continue intensive management.

Importantly, diabetes complications also have a significant psychosocial impact on patients' quality of life with negative outcomes for specific complications such as loss of independence, changes in occupational and family roles, increased social isolation with diabetic retinopathy, psychosocial difficulties with diabetic kidney disease, increased levels of depression, and anxiety in patients with lower limb amputations.[33,34] Furthermore, there is a significant and consistent association between depression and retinopathy, nephropathy, neuropathy, sexual dysfunction, and macrovascular complications, as well as an increased prevalence and odds for depression among patients with diabetes and other comorbid chronic diseases.[7,35]

Complications not only may exact a psychological toll but also may affect a patient's ability to engage in intensive management. Patients may begin to see themselves as handicapped or limited in their ability to carry out an intensive diabetes care regimen once complications are diagnosed. Perceived limitations may be physical or emotional. Onset of complications may be associated with a decline in optimism about treatment efficacy, resulting in less motivation to intensify efforts and reduced quality of life. Education regarding different treatment approaches and supports can renew the patient's commitment to achieving better glycemic control. Patients may need help understanding that any improvement in their glycemic status can improve their overall health status and delay the progression of complications. Healthcare professionals also should understand that distressing feelings in response to the diagnosis of complications are an expected and normal response; however, concerns may be warranted if a prolonged emotional response continues to interfere with patient's everyday functioning, and a referral to a mental health professional may be needed.

Coping and Problem-Solving Skills

Coping and problem-solving skills can be taught and practiced. Coping skills involve making prompt and effective changes to the diabetes care regimen when a problem arises. Peyrot and colleagues, in their biopsychosocial model of glycemic control in diabetes, explored the relationships among coping strategies, stress, and diabetes regimen adherence and found that people with T1D who used self-controlled coping (pragmatism and problem-solving) had better glycemic control and diabetes adherence than those who used emotional coping (anger, impulsive actions, anxious, and avoidant behaviors).[36] Furthermore, a study exploring patient–provider communication found that patients who used more self-controlled coping were less reluctant about discussing their self-care behaviors with providers.[37] Thus, it appears that efforts should be made to promote patients' pragmatic problem-solving approaches to diabetes distress.

Through problem-solving, individuals attempt to identify effective and adaptive solutions for specific problems encountered in everyday living. A review of the literature on problem-solving and diabetes found that problem-solving interventions demonstrated improvement in A1C for both children and adults and had a positive effect on psychosocial outcomes, such as reduced negative communication between parents and children or adolescents and improved self-efficacy in adults.[38] Effective diabetes-related coping and problem-solving include

- identifying factors that may contribute to adverse diabetes events (e.g., life stress; comorbidities; changes in insulin or technological devices, routine, eating, or exercise; and alcohol or medication use),
- recognizing one's ability and skills to evaluate the circumstances and respond appropriately, and
- informing and seeking support from a family member or healthcare professional who can help problem-solve and collaborate on treatment strategies and behaviors.

DIABETES MANAGEMENT

ADHERENCE SCREENING

Adherence is different than compliance. Rather than simple semantics, the difference implies a philosophy of treatment and expectations of the patients' and health professionals' roles. Compliance assumes an exact prescription for behavior and a hierarchy for treatment, which is counter to a patient-centered approach. With compliance, the provider knows best and the patient must comply with what the provider says without collaborating on the treatment regimen or treatment goals. Adherence assumes patient–clinician collaboration, which includes jointly defining problems, agreeing on specific problems, setting realistic treatment goals, and developing an action plan for achieving goals in the context of patient's life.

Systematic evaluation of adherence is unusual in clinical practice. In most cases, provider evaluation of patient adherence is subjective: partially based on the patients' report of what they have or haven't done, reports of adverse events such as hypoglycemia, and objective data such as A1C and weight. Interestingly, several studies have shown that some patients report reluctance to discuss their actual self-care behaviors with providers because of shame, guilt, and fear of judgment.[37,39,40] Therefore, it is not clear how much healthcare professionals actually learn about patients' self-care during treatment encounters. A trusting and nonjudgmental patient–clinician relationship may decrease patients' reluctance to discuss their self-care. Conducting a focused adherence screening in the

Table 4.1 — Practical Steps to Engage the Patient

Use a questionnaire or an interview to assess the following:

- Gaps in the patient's knowledge of diabetes and skills of diabetes self-care tasks
  - Administer a survey such as Self-Care Inventory–Revised (SCI-R)[41]
- Burden of self-care tasks
  - What is it like to live with these self-care tasks on a daily basis?
- Intentions regarding self-care behaviors
  - How do you intend to change and try this new self-care regimen?
- Attitudes about self-care changes
  - Explain the new self-care regimen. What is not clear?
  - How does the new self-care regimen address your goals for diabetes care?
  - Will this new self-care regimen have a positive effect on your diabetes? Why or why not?
  - How might this new self-care regimen be too difficult for you to do?
  - How might you be successful with this new self-care regimen?
- Self-efficacy
  - Why do you feel ready and able to follow this new self-care regimen?

Encourage patients to practice behavior in the following ways:

- Suggest the patient try a new self-care regimen or new technology.
- Meet more frequently with the patient to assess progress with self-care behaviors.

context of an effective relationship may allow the clinician to assess and develop patients' cooperation and skills so that together they can realistically develop the "best fit" treatment regimen. Some practical steps to engage the patient are listed in Table 4.1.

LIFESTYLE CHANGES

Many studies, including landmark trials Look AHEAD and U.K. Prospective Diabetes Study (UKPDS), have shown that lifestyle changes, particularly diet and exercise modification, must be implemented in addition to intensified self-care behaviors to achieve optimal metabolic control. As a result, the role of healthcare professionals has expanded to include helping patients initiate and maintain lifestyle changes that support intensive diabetes management. Behavioral strategies are used to achieve these goals within primary care and other medical settings.

Behavioral therapy within a context of social support has been shown to be effective in increasing exercise and modifying dietary intake, resulting in modest weight loss, improved glycemia, and reduced cardiac risk factors. Targeting and monitoring behavior change can be incorporated easily into routine diabetes care. Preliminary discussion of the behavior to be targeted and the goal to be achieved can occur while the physical examination takes place. This allows patients time to reflect on whether they are motivated to tackle changing a behavior at this particular time, consider whether the behavior change is realistic for them, and develop a feasible plan to implement the change. When instituting a behavioral program, the healthcare professional may develop an agreement with the patient, which may include the following steps:

1. Identify a behavior that the patient is willing to work to change (e.g., ask "Would you be willing to walk a half hour daily or eat two servings of vegetables daily?"), not one that is "prescribed."

2. Define the behavior in such a way that change can be monitored (e.g., have the patient keep a daily log of the activity).

3. Set a realistic goal for the change that you and the patient agree on (e.g., increase walking from zero times a week to three times a week for a half hour, *not* increase exercise from zero times a week to running 3 miles three times a week).

4. Establish and agree on the methods and supports necessary for the patient to change his or her daily routine (e.g., "What time of day would be convenient for this particular activity?").

5. Set a realistic date to accomplish the goal and for discussing the progress the patient has made using his or her written record.

6. If a routine checkup is not scheduled, arrange to communicate with the patient after 2 weeks regarding his or her progress, successes, and setbacks, during which time the patient and provider can identify barriers to success, generate problem-solving solutions, or modify the goal to make it either more manageable or challenging.

7. At the appointed follow-up visit or through electronic media, assess with the patient whether the new behavior has been mastered or more time is needed to make the behavior routine. If life circumstances have changed, more problem-solving may be needed, along with another plan for ensuring maintenance of the new behavior.

Once the agreement is made and documented (including significant others when appropriate), the provider can follow up by phone, fax, e-mail, or in person to monitor the intervention. Again, if patients are counseled that setbacks and difficulties are expected when changing lifestyle behaviors, a sense of failure can be attenuated if not prevented. Often, small changes in behavior not only improve the patient's medical outcome but also improve quality of life and enhance his or her feelings of efficacy and well-being.

PSYCHOSOCIAL SUPPORT SYSTEM

FAMILY SYSTEM

It is particularly important for the healthcare professional to assess the family system regarding attitudes toward intensification and medical care, willingness to participate in diabetes care, and financial resources. Family support is often a critical element in the success of intensive management because family members provide both concrete resources and emotional support for a patient's effort to improve his or her diabetes care. The process of intensifying treatment should be slowed and the healthcare professional should consider referral for counseling if family conflict around diabetes management is manifested. It is particularly important for the practitioner to assess the family system regarding attitudes toward intensification and medical care in general, willingness to participate in diabetes care, and financial resources. Conflicts can be avoided by having a clear discussion of diabetes care with all participating family members. This should specify who will take responsibility for which aspects of the regimen, the monitoring functions of each family member, and how the care regimen will or won't affect how the family lives. Attention is warranted when a patient reports being isolated and without a support system. This is especially important for emerging adults who have moved to a new city or for the elderly who live alone.

If motivation and commitment to intensive management come from a parent or a spouse, the relationship needs to be evaluated so that diabetes management does not become a vehicle for family conflict. It may become necessary to refer the patient and family for further diabetes education as well as interpersonal counseling. Family conflict over diabetes management can occur in any family when members disagree about treatment regimens, glycemic goals, and responsibilities of care. Families who are particularly susceptible are those with

- an adolescent patient whose wish for autonomy and independence from parental caretaking results in worsening glycemia,
- young children whose parents do not share the same strategies for self-care or goals,
- family members who perceive and express that the diabetes care routine negatively affects the family environment, or
- family members who feel that their needs are not being met because psychosocial and material resources are disproportionately expended on the family member with diabetes (this may apply to siblings as well as spouses).

Parents increasingly are seeking intensive treatment for their young children and adolescents with T1D or are initiating prevention efforts on behalf of their overweight children or adolescents who have prediabetes. Long-term concerns about the physical well-being of their child place an enormous burden on many parents. Thus, parents may have desires for an intensive treatment regimen that may not be feasible given the age and maturity of the child. Goals for treatment may not be shared by the child or adolescent and may excessively stress the family system. Issues of autonomy and decision-making regarding adherence to the prescribed treatment regimen also can lead to family conflict, regardless of the age of the patient. Decisions about the treatment regimen should be considered in the context of the patient's and family's wishes, adjustment to illness, resources, and abilities of all family members, especially when formulating regimens for children and adolescents. These caveats also apply to spousal systems and adult children taking care of elderly parents with diabetes.[42]

LIVING WITH OTHERS

Interpersonal support often contributes significantly to a patient's ability to implement and maintain intensive management. Psychosocial support can entail emotional support, which is nondirective and supplies a sense of caring and worth; tangible support, which is directive and offers concrete assistance; informational support, which includes guidance and help with problem-solving; and companionship support, which offers a sense of social belonging. Psychosocial support can help remove barriers to adherence because it eases the burden of illness; it can come from the whole healthcare team, a specific clinician, a family member, a religious leader or organization, or a diabetes support group.[32] Importantly, patients usually are most comfortable seeking support from people and institutions in cases in which they have established trusting relationships. Therefore, long-term continuity of care with healthcare professionals is an essential part of intensive management.

A patient's need for support varies depending on their individual characteristics and social networks. Healthcare professionals may facilitate patients seeking support by

- asking patients to identify individuals in their lives who would be willing to be educated to help with intensive diabetes management,
- including significant others in the planning of diabetes care regimens, and
- encouraging patients to share the responsibilities of diabetes care with family and friends to whatever extent they feel comfortable.

In addition, telemedicine visits or electronic media such as e-mail and text messages can replace phone calls or face-to-face meetings, allowing both patient and healthcare professional flexibility and ease of contact. As with other recommendations for care, establish frequency of communication so that expectations are clear between professionals and patients. In addition, ensure that Health Insurance Portability and Accountability Act regulations are observed and that a clear understanding develops between patient, support personnel, and providers regarding issues of privacy as well as who will be privy to information, particularly if underage children or adolescents are involved or if there are concerns for safety.

Intensified treatment may involve more public exposure of the patient's diabetes. For example, the patient may be less able to retire to a private location to more frequently check blood glucose or give an extra insulin bolus. Thus, intensive treatment may involve a patient coming to terms with the expectations and beliefs of others and needing to become his or her own patient advocate and educator. This may or may not feel comfortable to the individual, and the issue of private versus public business may need to be addressed and practiced. It is a common experience for people with diabetes to be asked, "Are you supposed to be eating that?" or, even more pointedly, to be told they are not supposed to be eating food with sugar. Having planned responses to these comments of "misguided helping" is part of living with diabetes. Anticipating such interactions is part of basic diabetes education, but this topic may need to be revisited during the process of intensification.

PATIENT–HEALTHCARE PROFESSIONAL RELATIONSHIP AND COMMUNICATION

Patient-centered medical treatment promotes physician–patient collaboration. Inherent to this collaboration are physicians' and patients' abilities to communicate effectively, develop a trusting interpersonal relationship, and discuss treatment-related decisions. Patients' active participation in the treatment team is another important part of the patient-centered approach. Patients, however, sometimes are afraid to tell their clinicians that they feel incapable of carrying out the requested behavior, are disinclined to do so because of fear or lack of resources, or disagree with the regimen prescription. Patients who do not feel a rapport with their clinicians are less likely to incorporate and sustain changes to their care regimen. Thus, establishing an atmosphere of collaboration and mutual respect during the treatment encounter will promote patients' cooperation. The collaborative physician–patient relationship in diabetes is associated with increased self-efficacy, improved attitudes toward diabetes and quality of life, decreased negative attitudes toward living with diabetes, and improved glycemic control.[39,43]

Patients' ability to discuss their self-care successes and difficulties with physicians enables physicians to individualize treatment prescriptions and recommendations, a necessary component of intensified treatment. Furthermore, physicians' ability to openly and effectively respond to patients' self-care reports, discuss immediate and long-term disease concerns, and provide treatment recommendations are important relationship and communication factors for optimal diabetes management. In a study exploring patient and physician perceptions of self-care communication, both physicians and patients recommended trust, nonjudgmental acceptance, open and honest communication, and providing patients hope for living with diabetes as important factors for improving self-care communication.[40] If trusting patient–clinician communication is established, patients may cope more easily with the demands of intensive management.

To promote patient involvement in diabetes management, it is important to

- include patients and their support system in the treatment team;
- collaborate on regimen, treatment goals, and self-care behaviors that are needed to achieve and maintain goals;
- adapt the regimen to the patient's lifestyle;
- have patients practice self-care behaviors;
- monitor the efficacy and outcomes of agreed-upon behaviors and redefine goals as necessary;
- renegotiate the treatment plan or behaviors if the current plan is not working; and, above all,
- stay positive, supportive, and nonjudgmental even when treatment goals are not being met.

HELPING PATIENTS WITH LONG-TERM ADHERENCE

Patient motivation, ability, and intention to maintain a complex regimen will vary over time. Choosing to focus less on diabetes care during periods of emotional turmoil, holidays, and vacation is to be expected. Other life events may temporarily take precedence over intensive diabetes management. By accepting that variation in self-management behaviors is expected (not aberrant), the healthcare professional can ensure that periodic lapses do not spiral into a sense of failure and frustration and disengagement from self-care. Some suggestions include the following: *1*) attempt to determine why the lapse in self-care behavior occurred, *2*) enlist the patient in making decisions regarding the redirection of treatment, and *3*) use a collaborative, nonjudgmental approach.

Intensification of diabetes management requires the patient to prioritize the diabetes care regimen. Note that treatment behaviors that have been mutually agreed on may not always result in the expected glycemic outcome. Factors such as stress, other disease processes, or changes in lifestyle or routine may affect glycemic control. Healthcare professionals and patients engaged in achieving optimal glycemia should not view unanticipated outcomes as failures of treatment. Instead, the patient and clinician can work to identify causal relationships between lifestyle, emotions, and glycemic status to develop self-care coping strategies. Healthcare professionals need to help patients understand that unexpected glycemic excursions should not be viewed as a personal failure, poor problem-solving, or treatment failure. The connection between new behaviors and glycemic control may not be immediate. Positive regard for small steps in behavior change may provide the support necessary until the patient's behavior becomes self-sustaining.

Helping patients formulate a regimen that is responsive to their lifestyles may ensure greater adherence with the prescribed treatment. A treatment regimen that fits into, rather than controls, lifestyle should be the goal of a sustainable treatment plan. When a patient is resistant to a healthcare professional's suggestions, nonadherence should not be assumed. A collaborative dialogue between patient and clinician can reestablish a working plan about self-management wherein the patient agrees to glycemic goals, and together strategies are developed that work toward resumption of intensive treatment goals.

CONCLUSION

Intensive diabetes management is presently the gold standard treatment for most patients with T1D and many patients with T2D who use insulin. Intensive treatment is challenging and patients may burn out, feel distressed, and have difficulties meeting these challenges. Patients can succeed when they are actively engaged in a collaborative patient–clinician relationship that is part of a multidisciplinary management strategy supported psychosocially by family, friends, coworkers, and members of their community. In addition, teaching and promoting patients' coping and problem-solving skills are critically important for improved management of the demanding tasks of intensive treatment as well as life stresses and lifestyle changes.

Active patient engagement requires that providers understand and address the psychosocial factors that may promote or interfere with patients performing or not performing the tasks of intensive diabetes management. Thus, a psychosocial assessment is essential to explore diabetes burnout, diabetes distress, depression, anxiety, eating disorders, and substance abuse, which are barriers to intensive management.

Importantly, patient–clinician collaboration highlights the need for patients to be actively engaged in their treatment. When providers respectfully inquire and listen for potential barriers to intensification, patients are able to set treatment goals that are responsive to their individual lifestyles. This increases the likelihood of successfully achieving these goals and may lessen patients' perceptions of the tasks of intensive treatment as an overwhelming burden.

Finally, patients and healthcare professionals need to understand and accept that long-term treatment adherence with intensive diabetes management may vary over time. Adherence depends on patients' psychological and physical status and reactions to life events and changes in lifestyle. A supportive treatment team with a trusting patient–healthcare professional relationship and communication can be a critical underpinning to patients' success in sustaining intensive diabetes management.

REFERENCES

1. Nathan DM, Zinman B, Cleary PA, et al. Modern-day clinical course of type 1 diabetes mellitus after 30 years' duration: the Diabetes Control and Complications Trial/Epidemiology of Diabetes Interventions and Complications and Pittsburgh Epidemiology of Diabetes Complications experience (1983–2005). *Arch Intern Med* 2009;169(14):1307–1316

2. Wing RR, Group LAR. Long-term effects of a lifestyle intervention on weight and cardiovascular risk factors in individuals with type 2 diabetes mellitus: four-year results of the Look AHEAD trial. *Arch Intern Med* 2010;170(17):1566–1575

3. Stetson B, Schlundt D, Peyrot M, et al. Monitoring in diabetes self-management: issues and recommendations for improvement. *Popul Health Manag* 2011;14(4):189–197

4. Welch GW, Jacobson AM, Polonsky WH. The problem areas in diabetes scale. An evaluation of its clinical utility. *Diabetes Care* 1997;20(5):760–766

5. Polonsky WH, Fisher L, Earles J, et al. Assessing psychosocial distress in diabetes: development of the Diabetes Distress Scale. *Diabetes Care* 2005;28(3):626–631

6. Kroenke K, Spitzer RL, Williams JB. The PHQ-9: validity of a brief depression severity measure. *J Gen Intern Med* 2001;16(9):606–613

7. Anderson RJ, Freedland KE, Clouse RE, Lustman PJ. The prevalence of comorbid depression in adults with diabetes: a meta-analysis. *Diabetes Care* 2001;24(6):1069–1078

8. Fisher L, Gonzalez JS, Polonsky WH. The confusing tale of depression and distress in patients with diabetes: a call for greater clarity and precision. *Diabet Med* 2014;31(7):764–772

9. Ducat L, Philipson LH, Anderson BJ. The mental health comorbidities of diabetes. *JAMA* 2014;312(7):691–692

10. American Diabetes Association. 12. Older adults: *Standards of Medical Care in Diabetes—2020. Diabetes Care* 2020;43(Suppl. 1):S152–S162

11. Anderson RJ, Grigsby AB, Freedland KE, et al. Anxiety and poor glycemic control: a meta-analytic review of the literature. *Int J Psychiatry Med* 2002;32(3):235–247

12. Anderbro T, Gonder-Frederick L, Bolinder J et al. Fear of hypoglycemia: relationship to hypoglycemic risk and psychological factors. *Acta Diabetol* 2015;52(3):581–589

13. Ritholz MD, Beste M, Edwards SS, et al. Impact of continuous glucose monitoring on diabetes management and marital relationships of adults with type 1 diabetes and their spouses: a qualitative study. *Diabet Med* 2014;31(1):47–54

14. Tamborlane WV, Beck RW, Bode BW, et al. Continuous glucose monitoring and intensive treatment of type 1 diabetes. *N Engl J Med* 2008;359(14): 1464–1476

15. Steenkamp D. Continuous glucose monitoring as a hypoglycemia mitigation tool in individuals with type 1 diabetes with impaired hypoglycemic awareness. *Endocr Pract* 2019;25(6):619–621

16. Brod M, Alolga SL, Meneghini L. Barriers to initiating insulin in type 2 diabetes patients: development of a new patient education tool to address myths, misconceptions and clinical realities. *Patient* 2014;7(4):437–450

17. Polonsky WH, Fisher L, Guzman S, Villa-Caballero L, Edelman SV. Psychological insulin resistance in patients with type 2 diabetes: the scope of the problem. *Diabetes Care* 2005;28(10):2543–2545

18. Rubin RR, Peyrot M. Psychological issues and treatments for people with diabetes. *J Clin Psychol* 2001;57(4):457–478

19. Jones JM, Lawson ML, Daneman D, Olmsted MP, Rodin G. Eating disorders in adolescent females with and without type 1 diabetes: cross sectional study. *BMJ* 2000;320(7249):1563–1566

20. Polonsky WH, Anderson BJ, Lohrer PA, et al. Insulin omission in women with IDDM. *Diabetes Care* 1994;17(10):1178–1185

21. Goebel-Fabbri AE, Fikkan J, Franko DL, et al. Insulin restriction and associated morbidity and mortality in women with type 1 diabetes. *Diabetes Care* 2008;31(3):415–419

22. Goebel-Fabbri AE, Anderson BJ, Fikkan J, et al. Improvement and emergence of insulin restriction in women with type 1 diabetes. *Diabetes Care* 2011;34(3):545–550

23. Markowitz JT, Butler DA, Volkening LK, et al. Brief screening tool for disordered eating in diabetes: internal consistency and external validity in a contemporary sample of pediatric patients with type 1 diabetes. *Diabetes Care* 2010;33(3):495–500

24. Zuijdwijk CS, Pardy SA, Dowden JJ, et al. The mSCOFF for screening disordered eating in pediatric type 1 diabetes. *Diabetes Care* 2014;37(2):e26–e27

25. de Zwaan M. Binge eating disorder and obesity. *Int J Obes Relat Metab Disord* 2001;25(Suppl. 1):S51–S55

26. Kenardy J, Mensch M, Bowen K, et al. Disordered eating behaviours in women with type 2 diabetes mellitus. *Eat Behav* 2001;2(2):183–192

27. Wilfley D, Berkowitz R, Goebel-Fabbri A, Hirst K, Ievers-Landis C, Lipman TH, et al. Binge eating, mood, and quality of life in youth with type 2 diabetes: baseline data from the TODAY Study. *Diabetes Care* 2011;34(4): 858–860

28. Young-Hyman DL, Davis CL. Disordered eating behavior in individuals with diabetes: importance of context, evaluation, and classification. *Diabetes Care* 2010;33(3):683–689

29. Ahmed AT, Karter AJ, Liu J. Alcohol consumption is inversely associated with adherence to diabetes self-care behaviours. *Diabet Med* 2006;23(7): 795–802

30. Weitzman ER, Ziemnik RE, Huang Q, Levy S. Alcohol and marijuana use and treatment nonadherence among medically vulnerable youth. *Pediatrics* 2015;136(3):450–457

31. Surwit RS, Schneider MS, Feinglos MN. Stress and diabetes mellitus. *Diabetes Care* 1992;15(10):1413–1422

32. Strom JL, Egede LE. The impact of social support on outcomes in adult patients with type 2 diabetes: a systematic review. *Curr Diab Rep* 2012;12(6): 769–781

33. Devenney R, O'Neill S. The experience of diabetic retinopathy: a qualitative study. *Br J Health Psychol* 2011;16(4):707–721

34. Coffey L, Gallagher P, Horgan O, Desmond D, MacLachlan M. Psychosocial adjustment to diabetes-related lower limb amputation. *Diabet Med* 2009;26(10):1063–1067

35. Egede LE. Effect of comorbid chronic diseases on prevalence and odds of depression in adults with diabetes. *Psychosom Med* 2005;67(1):46–51

36. Peyrot M, McMurry JF, Kruger DF. A biopsychosocial model of glycemic control in diabetes: stress, coping and regimen adherence. *J Health Soc Behav* 1999;40(2):141–158

37. Beverly EA, Ganda OP, Ritholz MD, et al. Look who's (not) talking: diabetic patients' willingness to discuss self-care with physicians. *Diabetes Care* 2012;35(7):1466–1472

38. Fitzpatrick SL, Schumann KP, Hill-Briggs F. Problem solving interventions for diabetes self-management and control: a systematic review of the literature. *Diabetes Res Clin Pract* 2013;100(2):145–161

39. Ciechanowski P, Katon WJ. The interpersonal experience of health care through the eyes of patients with diabetes. *Soc Sci Med* 2006;63(12): 3067–3079

40. Ritholz MD, Beverly EA, Brooks KM, Abrahamson MJ, Weinger K. Barriers and facilitators to self-care communication during medical appointments in the United States for adults with type 2 diabetes. *Chronic Illn* 2014;10(4): 303–313

41. Weinger K, Butler HA, Welch GW, La Greca AM. Measuring diabetes self-care: a psychometric analysis of the Self-Care Inventory–Revised with adults. *Diabetes Care* 2005;28(6):1346–1352

42. DiMatteo MR. Social support and patient adherence to medical treatment: a meta-analysis. *Health Psychol* 2004;23(2):207–218

43. Von Korff M, Gruman J, Schaefer J, Curry SJ, Wagner EH. Collaborative management of chronic illness. *Ann Intern Med* 1997;127(12):1097–1102

Patient Selection, Clinical Considerations, and Intensive Diabetes Management Goals

---

Highlights
Patient Selection, Clinical Considerations, and Intensive Diabetes Management Goals

- Appropriate patient selection is important when individualizing treatment regimens and goals of therapy.
- Patient characteristics that influence intensive diabetes management include
  - desire to improve glycemic management,
  - willingness to be actively involved in care,
  - access to adequate diabetes education,
  - ability to understand and implement a complex medical regimen,
  - ongoing, open communication with the healthcare team,
  - presence of adequate support networks.
- Treatment regimens often change over time to meet a patient's needs and balance risks and benefits, and regimens should be periodically reassessed and adjusted as needed.
- No single set of glycemic goals can be applied to every person with diabetes. Glycemic targets should be modified according to the patient's age, disease duration, type of diabetes, prior hypoglycemia history, lifestyle, diabetes complication status, concurrent medical conditions and support network.
- Intensive diabetes management is not feasible for all individuals, and best efforts should be made to encourage glycemic improvement in an individually appropriate and safe manner.

Patient Selection, Clinical Considerations, and Intensive Diabetes Management Goals

Intensive diabetes management has been associated with improved long-term diabetes outcomes, but it is not necessarily appropriate, or achievable, for all patients. Successful intensive diabetes management incorporates diabetes self-management principles and strategies along with a set of intensive glycemic targets. The efficacy of intensive management is influenced by individual patient characteristics, as well as the efforts of his or her healthcare team. Intensive diabetes therapy consists of insulin therapy, either basal-bolus insulin replacement using multiple daily injections, or continuous subcutaneous insulin infusion pumps with or without continuous glucose monitoring (CGM) augmentation, for patients with type 1 diabetes (T1D), but it may also involve noninsulin therapies for those with type 2 diabetes (T2D). Given recent advances in diabetes pharmacotherapy, many patients with T2D may now be able to achieve intensive glycemic goals with medications that minimize hypoglycemia, and therefore, certain patient selection criteria discussed in this chapter, including hypoglycemia risk, may not be as relevant in this population. This chapter will focus on appropriate patient selection for intensive diabetes management and glycemic targets, as well as special scenarios where these targets may differ.

RECOMMENDED GLYCEMIC TARGETS

Although diabetes care must be individualized, the goal for most patients is to pursue glycemic targets that are as close to normal as safely possible. Glycemic targets for fingerstick blood glucose monitoring and glycated hemoglobin A_{1c} (A1C) have been refined over the last several decades, and additional targets using CGM data are also now available (see Table 5.1). International consensus with regard to CGM metrics suggests that clinicians consider using the ambulatory glucose profile (AGP) as a standard metric, incorporating a minimum of 70% of sensor-derived glucose data over a 14-day period in their evaluation of glycemic goals.[1,2] However, all of the currently available targets do not specifically incorporate or isolate assessment and recommendations with regard to overnight glucose levels, where targets often need to be higher to prevent nocturnal hypoglycemia.

Table 5.1 — Guidelines for Intensive Management Targets

Many nonpregnant adults

Glycated hemoglobin A_{1c}	<7% (53 mmol/mol)*
Preprandial capillary plasma glucose	80–130 mg/dL (4.4–7.2 mmol/L)
Peak postprandial capillary plasma glucose	<180 mg/dL (<10.0 mmol/L)**

Postprandial glucose should be targeted if A1C goals are not met despite achievement of preprandial glucose goals.**
CGM time in range 70–180 mg/dL (3.9–10 mmol/L) >70% (>16 h, 48 min)
CGM time below range <70 mg/dL (3.9 mmol/L) <4% (<1 h)
CGM time below range <54 mg/dL (3.0 mmol/L) <1% (<15 min)
CGM time above range >180 mg/dL (10.0 mmol/L) <25% (<6 h)
CGM time above range >250 mg/dL (13.9 mmol/L) <5% (<1 h, 12 min)

Conception and pregnancy

A1C ideally <6.5% (48 mmol/mol) during preconception
A1C ideally <6% during pregnancy

Preprandial capillary blood glucose	<95 mg/dL (5.3 mmol/L)
and either:	
1-h postprandial capillary blood glucose	<140 mg/dL (7.8 mmol/L)
or	
2-h postprandial capillary blood glucose	<120 mg/dL (6.7 mmol/L)

CGM time in range 63–140 mg/dL (3.5–7.8 mmol/L) >70% (>16 h, 48 min)***
CGM time below range <63 mg/dL (3.5 mmol/L) <4% (<1 h)***
CGM time below range <54 mg/dL (3.0 mmol/L) <1% (<15 min)***
CGM time above range >140 mg/dL (7.8 mmol/L) <25% (<6 h)***

*Referenced to a nondiabetic range of 4.0–6.0% using a Diabetes Control and Complications Trial (DCCT)-based assay.
**Postprandial glucose measurements should be performed 1–2 h after the beginning of the meal.
***CGM recommendations only for pregnant women with T1D, not for T2D or gestational diabetes.

PATIENT SELECTION AND CLINICAL CONSIDERATIONS

When setting glycemic targets, the goals of intensive diabetes management must be individualized using a collaborative process of shared decision-making between the patient and the healthcare team. Patients should be encouraged and supported to reach the most intensive glucose goals they are capable of safely achieving, but these targets may also change over time and should be readdressed frequently.

Patients should be educated on what intensive glycemic control entails, including the risks and benefits, because the decision to pursue intensive glycemic control is ultimately up to the patient. The benefits of intensive glycemic control for prevention and reduction in progression of microvascular complications are well documented.[3,4] Cardiovascular benefits have also been reported for patients with T1D managed with intensive glycemic control, but similar benefits are not consistently reported in those with long-standing T2D or for those at high risk for cardiovascular disease. Mortality may actually increase with intensive glycemic management in these populations.[5,6]

Discussions about the potential benefits of intensive glucose management should be ongoing, and glycemic targets should be adjusted over time. In addition, exploration of patient feelings and concerns about diabetes management is a key component of forming a therapeutic alliance and may facilitate intensification of management over time. Clinicians should be sensitive to the potential challenges of keeping up with the rigorous demands of an intensive diabetes regimen. Factors to consider include the patient's age, interpersonal support, and general health status. Socioeconomic status also may play a role in the feasibility of intensive regimens.

- Is the patient cognitively and emotionally capable of assuming primary responsibility for daily diabetes care and treatment decisions?
- If not, is there a responsible individual who is willing to be educated and to actively participate in a complex regimen for the patient?
- If the patient lives alone, who will have daily or frequent contact with the patient in case of emergencies, such as severe hypoglycemia or illness requiring outside intervention?
- Does the patient's home, work, or academic environment permit and support the behaviors needed for intensive treatment?
- Does the patient have the financial resources to pay for the increased costs associated with intensive treatment?

Tailoring care to specific patient needs and taking into account these factors is more likely to result in success compared to a generalized approach to care. Regular contact between the patient and healthcare team increases the likelihood of success with intensive management, particularly because the healthcare team often extends beyond the diabetologist to include diabetes educators, nurses, pharmacists, and dietitians. Although medical management is the backbone of intensive management, a comprehensive approach to care is necessary to optimize diabetes care and can affect quality of life more than just glucose control.

Intensive diabetes management should be considered for most individuals with T1D. Indeed, it is the current and standard medical treatment for the disease. The lowest targets that can safely be achieved without increasing hypoglycemia are recommended for most patients. This is particularly true for

- motivated individuals with no early evidence of complications,
- women who are pregnant or contemplating pregnancy, and
- individuals with newly diagnosed diabetes.

Caution should be exercised when deciding whether to pursue intensive treatment for specific patient groups that are at higher risk for complications (see Table 5.2). In some cases, although there may be clear benefits, they may not outweigh the potential risks.

Table 5.2—Patient Characteristics That Influence the Treatment Goals and Feasibility of Intensive Diabetes Management

- Hypoglycemia unawareness
- A history of recurrent severe hypoglycemic episodes
- Use of medications that may interfere with hypoglycemia detection or treatment (e.g., β-blockers)
- Other medical conditions that can be aggravated by hypoglycemia (e.g., cerebrovascular disease or angina)
- Severe psychiatric disorders, impaired cognitive ability, or psychosocial stressors
- Alcohol or substance abuse disorders
- Advanced end-stage diabetes complications
- Cardiovascular disease and longer duration T2D
- Symptomatic coronary artery disease
- Cardiac arrhythmias
- Concurrent diseases or conditions that would functionally limit intensive management (e.g., debilitating arthritis or severe visual impairment)
- Relatively short life expectancy

PATIENTS WITH TYPE 2 DIABETES

Intensive diabetes management should not be restricted to those with T1D but should also be considered for most individuals with T2D. Treatment for T2D may include insulin therapy, but it may also consist of noninsulin therapies used in combination with each other or with insulin. The tenets of diabetes management are similar for both types of diabetes, namely frequent blood glucose monitoring, medication compliance, dietary modification, regular physical activity, and ongoing communication with the healthcare team.

Lowering blood glucose levels toward the normal range is desirable to decrease risk of complications, especially in those with shorter duration of diabetes or in the absence of existing cardiovascular disease.[5] If this can be accomplished by regimens involving nutritional counseling, physical activity, healthy weight loss, and oral or injected noninsulin glucose-lowering agents, then a more intensive insulin regimen may not be necessary. Treatment options that are weight neutral or that have modest associated weight loss should be considered first. Medical management should be further individualized, taking into consideration comorbid risk factors, such as the presence of cardiovascular or kidney disease. Certain evidence-based noninsulin therapies, such as glucagon-like peptide 1 receptor agonists (GLP-1RA) or sodium–glucose cotransporter 2 (SGLT2) inhibitors, have been proven to improve important cardiovascular and kidney outcomes in T2D and may be preferred over insulin, at least initially.[7,8] However, β-cell function is expected to decline over time as the disease progresses, and insulin replacement therapy may be necessary and should not be delayed when indicated.

HYPOGLYCEMIA

One of the principal limiting factors in achieving intensive diabetes management goals is the increased risk of hypoglycemia that is particularly relevant for patients using insulin therapy. The advent of and widespread growth in the use of CGM has greatly enhanced our understanding of hypoglycemia and has allowed us to define and recognize hypoglycemia with greater clarity than in the past. Level 1 hypoglycemia is defined as a glucose level between 54 and 70 mg/dL, level 2 hypoglycemia is a glucose level <54 mg/dL, and level 3 hypoglycemia is a hypoglycemic event requiring assistance for treatment.[9] With intensive diabetes management, episodes of level 1 hypoglycemia are expected and may be less clinically meaningful than was previously recognized; as long as time spent in this low range is minimized (<60 min/day), symptoms are recognized, treated, and do not interfere with daily life or present any danger to the patient or others. In fact, CGM-derived normative data have shown that most healthy individuals without diabetes have some sensor glucose values that fall within the level 1 hypoglycemic range.[10] However, many diabetes therapies induce hypoglycemia, and if there is risk of harm from hypoglycemia, then the etiology of the hypoglycemia must be explored and, if necessary, glycemic targets must be raised to mitigate this risk. Factors to consider when establishing treatment goals and to minimize risk of hypoglycemia are listed in Table 5.3.

Beyond the day-to-day risk of hypoglycemic episodes, recurrent hypoglycemia has been associated with increased rates of hypoglycemic unawareness, dementia, and increased mortality in adults, so minimization of hypoglycemia is essential even while strict glycemic targets are pursued.[5,11] Although hypoglycemia

Table 5.3—Factors to Consider When Establishing Individualized Treatment Goals

- Age
- Type of diabetes (type 1, type 2, or gestational)
- Duration of diabetes
- Presence and severity of diabetes complications
- Presence of other medical conditions or treatments that might alter the response to therapy or prevent the patient from carrying out self-care behaviors
- Ability and desire of patient to understand and implement a complex treatment regimen
- History of repeated, severe hypoglycemia
- Ability to recognize hypoglycemic symptoms (hypoglycemia unawareness)
- Lifestyle and occupation (e.g., possible risks of experiencing hypoglycemia on the job)
- Financial constraints
- Level of support available from family and friends
- Willingness to be actively involved in daily diabetes management
- Skill in diabetes self-management techniques
- Awareness and acceptance of benefits and risks associated with intensive management
- Ongoing connection and communication with the healthcare team

unawareness was previously considered an absolute contraindication to intensive diabetes management, this is no longer the case. Use of continuous glucose monitors as adjuncts to intensive insulin therapy (in multiple-dose insulin [MDI] and pump users) has been associated with a reduction in hypoglycemia through a variety of increasingly automated functions, including use of predictive CGM hypoglycemia alerts, automated suspension of basal insulin delivery when hypoglycemia is predicted to occur within the next 30 min, and basal insulin attenuation algorithms incorporated into currently available hybrid closed-loop insulin pump systems.[12,13] In patients who have been identified as having hypoglycemia unawareness, avoidance of hypoglycemia for 2–4 weeks has been associated with reversal of hypoglycemia unawareness and return of protective symptoms.[14]

GOAL-SETTING FOR SPECIAL POPULATIONS

No single set of blood glucose targets can be applied to every person with diabetes, and glycemic targets should be individualized. The following sections further explore glycemic targets in specific populations in which different glycemic targets may be appropriate.

PREGNANCY

A lower glycemic target range is recommended during pregnancy because lower blood glucose levels have been associated with improved pregnancy outcomes.[15] The American Diabetes Association recommends monitoring of fasting and postprandial glucose levels for most pregnant women, but for those on full insulin replacement therapy or insulin pump therapy, preprandial glucose monitoring is also recommended.[1] The current recommendations are preprandial fasting glucose levels <95 mg/dL (5.30 mmol/L) and either 1-h postprandial glucose levels <140 mg/dL (7.8 mmol/L) or 2-h postprandial glucose levels of <120 mg/dL (6.7 mmol/L). Achieving these targets requires more effort on the part of the patient and the healthcare team, as well as frequent communication and active support. Avoidance of recurrent or severe hypoglycemia must be considered in the pursuit of these stringent glycemic goals.

A1C levels fall naturally during pregnancy due to increased red blood cell turnover, and A1C is typically considered a secondary measure of glycemic control in pregnancy after fingerstick blood glucose monitoring.[1] Depending on the risk of maternal hypoglycemia, A1C targets should be lower and aim for ranges as close to normal during pregnancy. There are increasing data to support the use of CGM during pregnancy, particularly to mitigate the risk of hypoglycemia while simultaneously targeting lower glucose levels.[16] For women with T1D, it is recommended that the following CGM targets be set: >70% time in range 63–140 mg/dL (3.5–7.8 mmol/L), <4% below range <63 mg/dL (3.5 mmol/L), and <25% above range >140 mg/dL (7.8 mmol/L).[2] Due to insufficient data, there are no current recommendations for CGM targets in pregnant women with T2D or gestational diabetes.

CHILDREN

Although glycemic targets for children historically have focused on those with T1D, increasing rates of childhood-onset T2D have led to a need to differentiate care goals between these groups and promote setting of individualized glycemic targets. The American Diabetes Association released position statements on the management of both T1D and T2D in 2018 to address these differences.[17,18] Children require a team with special expertise and experience in the management of childhood diabetes. When such a team is available, intensive diabetes management is encouraged.

The goal in children with T1D is to lower glucose while mitigating the risk of hypoglycemia through intensive insulin management, either multiple daily injections or continuous subcutaneous insulin infusion.[17] The patient's history of severe hypoglycemia and associated neurological and neuropsychological risk needs to be carefully considered when setting individualized glycemic targets for children with T1D. Young children <6–7 years old are particularly vulnerable to the long-term adverse effects of severe or repeated hypoglycemia and may not be able to recognize or manage hypoglycemia when it occurs.[19] Automated insulin delivery systems and CGM should be considered for all children and adolescents with T1D while paying particular attention to adherence and ongoing use of the devices. Although glycemic targets for young children had been higher in the past, in concert with the availability and rapid growth in the use of continuous glucose monitoring in children, an A1C level of <7% is appropriate for many children. This target should be individualized depending on individual factors and more stringent targets may be appropriate if they can be achieved safely.[17] Lower A1C targets have been associated with lower rates of microvascular and macrovascular complications in children with diabetes, and an A1C level of 6.5% may be appropriate in some cases.[20]

In children and adolescents with T2D, an A1C target of <7% is typically recommended for most patients.[18] Rates of hypoglycemia in children and adolescents with T2D are quite low, particularly among those on oral medications only, so lower targets may be achievable.[21]

OLDER ADULT PATIENTS

Glycemic targets in older adult patients (age >65 years) warrant special consideration. Older adults with diabetes more commonly have coexisting medical conditions, such as cognitive dysfunction, depression, risk of falls, and chronic pain, in addition to polypharmacy.[22] These issues may interfere with patients' abilities to perform self-care tasks, such as blood glucose monitoring, following complex medication regimens, and adhering to recommended diet and exercise regimens.[23] In addition, older adults are often reluctant to make changes in their insulin doses between clinic visits or during illness. Avoidance of hypoglycemia and malnutrition is a priority in older patients, and loosening of glycemic targets to achieve this is often appropriate in certain patients (history of dementia, cognitive impairment, history of severe hypoglycemia, limited life expectancy).

In otherwise healthy older adults with few comorbidities, an A1C goal of <7.0–7.5% may be appropriate, whereas in those with multiple comorbidities or those at higher risk for severe hypoglycemia, a target of <8.0–8.5% may be reasonable.[24] In some very frail individuals, the glycemic goals may be even further limited to avoid severe hyperglycemia, which may increase the risk of nocturia or urinary incontinence, infections, dehydration, decubitus ulcers, and other consequences of catabolism associated with hyperglycemia. Older individuals should be reassessed over time for changes in clinical status to allow for adjustment of glycemic targets to minimize risk of hypoglycemia.

CONCLUSION

Intensive glycemic management should be encouraged for patients who are motivated to achieve the lowest glycemic levels safely possible. The benefits of intensive glucose management must always be considered in the context of the potential risks, particularly the increased risk of hypoglycemia. Glucose targets should be individualized in each patient. These targets should be reassessed over time to ensure that they are still appropriate. If treatment strategies are to be effective in reducing long-term sequelae, then treatment goals and implementation techniques must be sustained over time. Inability to reach the ideal glycemic target should not be viewed as a treatment failure or a patient failure. It is essential for the patient to have a strong relationship with his or her healthcare team to increase the likelihood of success with the increased demands of intensive glycemic control. No patient should be dismissed arbitrarily as ineligible or unsuitable for intensified diabetes management efforts, and all patients should be educated about the risks and benefits to best individualize their care and be provided with the requisite knowledge, skills, and resources to allow them to succeed.

REFERENCES

1. American Diabetes Association. Summary of revisions: *Standards of Medical Care in Diabetes—2020. Diabetes Care* 2020;43(Suppl. 1):S4–S6

2. Battelino T, Danne T, Bergenstal RM, et al. Clinical targets for continuous glucose monitoring data interpretation: recommendations from the International Consensus on Time in Range. *Diabetes Care* 2019;42(8):1593–1603

3. Nathan DM, Genuth S, Lachin J, et al. The effect of intensive treatment of diabetes on the development and progression of long-term complications in insulin-dependent diabetes mellitus. *N Engl J Med* 1993;329(14):977–986

4. UK Prospective Diabetes Study (UKPDS) Group. Intensive blood-glucose control with sulphonylureas or insulin compared with conventional treatment and risk of complications in patients with type 2 diabetes (UKPDS 33). *Lancet* 1998;352(9131):837–853

5. Gerstein HC, Miller ME, Byington RP, et al. Effects of intensive glucose lowering in type 2 diabetes. *N Engl J Med* 2008;358(24):2545–2559

6. Skyler JS, Bergenstal R, Bonow RO, et al. Intensive glycemic control and the prevention of cardiovascular events: implications of the ACCORD, ADVANCE, and VA diabetes trials: a position statement of the American Diabetes Association and a scientific statement of the American College of Cardiology Foundation and the American Heart Association. *Diabetes Care* 2009;32(1):187–192

7. Marso SP, Daniels GH, Brown-Frandsen K, et al. Liraglutide and cardiovascular outcomes in type 2 diabetes. *N Engl J Med* 2016;375(4):311–322

8. Zelniker TA, Wiviott SD, Raz I, et al. SGLT2 inhibitors for primary and secondary prevention of cardiovascular and renal outcomes in type 2 diabetes: a systematic review and meta-analysis of cardiovascular outcome trials. *Lancet* 2019;393(10166):31–39

9. Agiostratidou G, Anhalt H, Ball D, et al. Standardizing clinically meaningful outcome measures beyond HbA1c for type 1 diabetes: a consensus report of the American Association of Clinical Endocrinologists, the American Association of Diabetes Educators, the American Diabetes Association, the Endocrine Society, JDRF International, the Leona M. and Harry B. Helmsley Charitable Trust, the Pediatric Endocrine Society, and the T1D Exchange. *Diabetes Care* 2017;40(12):1622–1630

10. Shah VN, DuBose SN, Li Z, et al. Continuous glucose monitoring profiles in healthy nondiabetic participants: a multicenter prospective study. *J Clin Endocrinol Metab* 2019;104(10):4356–4364

11. Whitmer RA, Karter AJ, Yaffe K, Quesenberry CP, Selby JV. Hypoglycemic episodes and risk of dementia in older patients with type 2 diabetes mellitus. *JAMA* 2009;301(15):1565–1572

12. Heinemann L, Freckmann G, Ehrmann D, et al. Real-time continuous glucose monitoring in adults with type 1 diabetes and impaired hypoglycaemia awareness or severe hypoglycaemia treated with multiple daily insulin injections (HypoDE): a multicentre, randomised controlled trial. *Lancet* 2018;391(10128):1367–1377

13. Brown SA, Kovatchev BP, Raghinaru D, et al. Six-month randomized, multicenter trial of closed-loop control in type 1 diabetes. *N Engl J Med* 2019;381(18):1707–1717

14. Cryer PE, Davis SN, Shamoon H. Hypoglycemia in diabetes. *Diabetes Care* 2003;26(6):1902–1912

15. Metzger BE, Lowe LP, Dyer AR, et al. Hyperglycemia and adverse pregnancy outcomes. *N Engl J Med* 2008;358(19):1991–2002

16. Feig DS, Donovan LE, Corcoy R, et al. Continuous glucose monitoring in pregnant women with type 1 diabetes (CONCEPTT): a multicentre international randomised controlled trial. *Lancet* 2017;390(10110):2347–2359

17. Chiang JL, Maahs DM, Garvey KC, et al. Type 1 diabetes in children and adolescents: a position statement by the American Diabetes Association. *Diabetes Care* 2018;41(9):2026–2044

18. Arslanian S, Bacha F, Grey M, et al. Evaluation and management of youth-onset type 2 diabetes: a position statement by the American Diabetes Association. *Diabetes Care* 2018;41(12):2648–2668

19. Abraham MB, Jones TW, Naranjo D, et al. ISPAD Clinical Practice Consensus Guidelines 2018: assessment and management of hypoglycemia in children and adolescents with diabetes. *Pediatr Diabetes* 2018;19(Suppl. 27): 178–192

20. Diabetes Control and Complications Trial Research Group. Effect of intensive diabetes treatment on the development and progression of long-term complications in adolescents with insulin-dependent diabetes mellitus: Diabetes Control and Complications Trial. *J Pediatr* 1994;125(2):177–188

21. TODAY Study Group. Safety and tolerability of the treatment of youth-onset type 2 diabetes: the TODAY experience. *Diabetes Care* 2013;36(6):1765–1771

22. Kimbro LB, Mangione CM, Steers WN, et al. Depression and all-cause mortality in persons with diabetes mellitus: are older adults at higher risk? Results from the Translating Research Into Action for Diabetes Study. *J Am Geriatr Soc* 2014;62(6):1017–1022

23. Kirkman MS, Briscoe VJ, Clark N, et al. Diabetes in older adults. *Diabetes Care* 2012;35(12):2650–2664

24. Laiteerapong N, Iveniuk J, John PM, Laumann EO, Huang ES. Classification of older adults who have diabetes by comorbid conditions, United States, 2005–2006. *Prev Chronic Dis* 2012;9:E100

Multicomponent Insulin Regimens

Highlights
Multicomponent
Insulin Regimens

- Multicomponent insulin regimens typically use two out of six available types of insulin:
  - Ultra-rapid-acting mealtime insulins currently include fast-acting insulin aspart (Fiasp), fast-acting insulin lispro (Lyumjev), and insulin human inhalation powder, allowing for injection or inhalation of insulin prior to or immediately after meals.
  - Following the ultra-rapid-acting insulins, the rapid-acting human insulin analogs lispro, aspart, and glulisine have the most rapid onset of action and time to peak effect and the shortest duration of action.
  - The short-acting insulin (regular insulin) is a less commonly prescribed mealtime insulin; however, it is a viable option for those who cannot afford insulin analogs.
  - The intermediate-acting insulin (NPH insulin; also called isophane) has a more delayed onset of action and peak effect and a longer duration of action. NPH insulin is more affordable than long-acting insulin analogs and can be used twice daily for basal insulin needs.
  - The long-acting analog insulins U-100 glargine and detemir have relatively long duration action profiles and are nearly peakless.
  - The ultra-long-acting analog insulins degludec and U-300 glargine have even longer action profiles than U-100 glargine and detemir and are peakless.
- Insulin absorption and availability are influenced by
  - anatomical regions of injections, with the fastest absorption from the abdomen and the slowest from the thigh (specific to regular, NPH, and mixed insulins containing NPH);
  - timing of premeal injections;
  - factors such as exercise, showering, bathing, and ambient temperature; and
  - injection of insulin into areas of lipoatrophy, scarring, and lipohypertrophy.
- Multicomponent insulin regimens attempt to mimic physiological insulin release.
  - These regimens consist of various combinations of basal and prandial insulin components.
  - Frequent self-monitoring of blood glucose and/or continuous glucose monitoring guide appropriate changes in insulin dosage and timing, food intake, and activity profile.

- Prandial insulin is administered by injection using a syringe, pen, or alternatively as a continuous infusion through an insulin pump, or inhaled in the case of insulin human inhalation powder.
- Basal insulin is either administered utilizing a rapid-acting analog via insulin pump or via injection using an insulin pen or syringe.

■ Specific insulin regimens allow individual, flexible combinations of insulins and analogs that are suitable for various lifestyles, including

- premeal ultra-rapid-acting (fast-acting insulin analog or insulin human inhalation powder) or rapid-acting (lispro, aspart, or glulisine) or short-acting (regular insulin) and basal glargine, detemir, or degludec;
- premeal ultra-rapid-acting (fast-acting insulin analog or insulin human inhalation powder) or rapid-acting (lispro, aspart, or glulisine) or short-acting (regular insulin) and basal NPH; and
- continuous subcutaneous insulin infusion of rapid-acting, ultra-rapid-acting or, rarely, buffered regular human insulin.

■ Other insulin regimens that offer less flexibility and generally less intensive management options are

- twice-daily mixtures of regular or rapid-acting insulin and NPH;
- prebreakfast rapid-acting, or regular insulin and NPH, predinner rapid-acting or regular insulin, and bedtime NPH;

■ Total daily insulin dosages are typically calculated based on body weight (wt) and usually range from 0.2 to 1 unit/kg body wt/day. Dosage requirements vary considerably during the remission or "honeymoon" phase of type 1 diabetes (when there is residual β-cell function), intercurrent illness, adolescence, or pregnancy.

■ Total daily insulin dosage is then divided into basal and prandial components:

- Basal insulin typically accounts for 40–50% of the total daily dose.
- The remainder is divided among the meals, using insulin-to-carbohydrate ratios or preset dose guidelines.
- All regimens must be individualized according to the patient's desires, lifestyle, age, comorbidities, concomitant medications, and defined target level of glycemic control.

■ Insulin adjustments consist of an action plan for the alteration of therapy to achieve individually defined glycemic goals.

- Changes are made in insulin dosage, timing of injections, or the meal plan guided by self-monitoring of blood glucose and/or continuous glucose monitoring results.
- Pattern adjustments consist of modification of the current insulin dosage to minimize glycemic excursions throughout the day and to avoid hypoglycemia (<70 mg/dL).

Multicomponent Insulin Regimens

This chapter discusses the design and use of insulin regimens for intensive diabetes management.

INSULIN TIMING AND ACTION

There are six general categories of time course of insulin action:

- ultra-rapid-acting insulin (e.g., fast-acting insulin analogs [Fiasp, fast-acting insulin lispro] and insulin human inhalation powder),
- rapid-acting insulin (e.g., insulin lispro, aspart, and glulisine [genetically engineered insulin analogs]),
- short-acting insulin (e.g., regular [soluble]),
- intermediate-acting insulin (NPH, isophane),
- long-acting insulin (U-100 glargine and detemir [genetically engineered insulin analogs]), and
- ultra-long-acting insulin (degludec and U-300 glargine [genetically engineered insulin analogs]).

Table 6.1 summarizes the nominal action profiles—time to peak action and duration of action—of these insulin preparations.

Two general pharmacokinetic principles apply: First, a longer time to peak results in a broader peak and longer duration of action. Second, with increasing insulin dose, the breadth of the peak and the duration of action tend to be somewhat lengthened. The values included in Table 6.1 are for doses of 10–15 units, or 0.1–0.2 unit/kg.

Ultra-Rapid-Acting Insulin

Faster-acting insulin aspart (Fiasp) is conventional insulin aspart combined with niacinamide (vitamin B3), which helps accelerate absorption of insulin into subcutaneous capillaries, and L-arginine, which helps stabilize the formulation.[1] Fiasp can be injected immediately prior to a meal and has shown comparative efficacy to premeal insulin aspart when injected up to 20 min into (immediately after) a meal.[2] Faster-acting insulin lispro (Lyumjev) is conventional insulin lispro with additions of treprostinil to facilitate local vasodilation and sodium

Table 6.1 — Insulins by Comparative Action

	Onset	Peak action	Effective duration
Ultra-rapid-acting			
Fast-acting insulin aspart (analog)[†]	2–15 min	90–120 min	5–7 h
Fast-acting insulin lispro (analog)[‡]	2–15 min	40–60 min	5–7 h
Insulin human inhalation powder	12 min	30–60 min	1.5–4.5 h
Rapid-acting			
Insulin lispro (analog)	5–15 min	30–90 min	3–5 h
Insulin aspart (analog)	5–15 min	30–90 min	3–5 h
Insulin glulisine (analog)	5–15 min	30–90 min	3–5 h
Short-acting			
Regular (soluble)	30–60 min	2–3 h	5–8 h
Intermediate-acting			
NPH (isophane)	2–4 h	4–10 h	10–16 h
Long-acting			
Insulin glargine U-100 (analog)	2–4 h	Peakless	20–24 h
Insulin detemir (analog)	2–4 h	6–14 h	16–20 h
Ultra-long-acting			
Insulin glargine U-300 (analog)	6 h	Peakless	Up to 36 h
Insulin degludec (analog)	30–90 min	Peakless	24–42 h
Combinations			
70% degludec, 30% aspart	5–15 min	Dual	24–42 h
70% NPH, 30% regular	30–60 min	Dual	12–18 h
70% NPA,[‡] 30% aspart	5–15 min	Dual	12–18 h
75% NPL,[¶] 25% lispro	5–15 min	Dual	12–18 h
50% NPL, 50% lispro	5–15 min	Dual	12–18 h

[†]Onset of action shown to be ~5 min faster than conventional insulin aspart; peak action shown to be 7.3 min faster than conventional insulin aspart.[3]
[‡]Compared to insulin lispro, time of onset of action reduced by 27%, and duration of action decreased by 68 min[4]; time to reach half-maximal drug concentration ~6 min faster than fast-acting insulin aspart, and ~12 min faster than conventional insulin lispro.[5]
[‡]Neutral protamine aspart.
[¶]Neutral protamine lispro.

citrate to improve absorption into capillaries, thus speeding onset of action.[4] Similar to Fiasp, Lyumjev can also be injected immediately prior to a meal or 20 min into (immediately after) a meal. In a phase 3 study, Lyumjev demonstrated noninferiority in hemoglobin A_{1c} (A1C) reduction and superiority to insulin lispro in controlling 1- and 2-h postprandial hyperglycemia.[6] Faster-acting insulin lispro demonstrated faster absorption time when compared to faster-acting insulin aspart and conventional insulin lispro. It took 13 min for faster-acting lispro to reach half-maximal drug concentration, compared to 19 min for faster-acting aspart and 25 min for insulin lispro (Fig. 6.1).[5] In a separate study comparing faster-acting insulin lispro with conventional insulin lispro, time of onset was decreased by 27%, 6.4 min as compared to 11 min, and total duration of action was shorter, decreased by 68 min.[4] Given the formulation changes to the faster-acting analogs, they have the potential to more closely mimic physiologic insulin release and action as compared with rapid-acting insulin analogs.[7] They have demonstrated improved coverage of postmeal glucose excursions, leading to modestly improved peak postprandial blood glucose, which can result in improved A1C.[2,7–9]

Insulin human inhalation powder is human regular insulin formulated with fumaryl diketopiperazine (FDKP) and absorbed onto technosphere particles. FDKP forms a crystalline structure at acidic pH, allowing for inhalation of the microparticles. FDKP becomes rapidly soluble at neutral or basic pH, and once inhaled and reaching physiologic pH inside lung tissue, it quickly solubilizes and releases the insulin for rapid absorption into capillaries.[10,11] Once in the circulation, the pharmacokinetics (PK) follows that of human insulin, with faster onset of action due to rapid pulmonary absorption, thus allowing for usage at the beginning of meals (Figue 6.2).[12] In studies, insulin human inhalation powder has been reported to result in noninferior reduction of A1C in patients with type 1 diabetes (T1D) and has been reported to contribute to decreased hypoglycemia and weight gain as compared to injectable insulin aspart, but with the risk of increased cough.[10] Inhaled insulin should not be used in patients with chronic lung disease.[11]

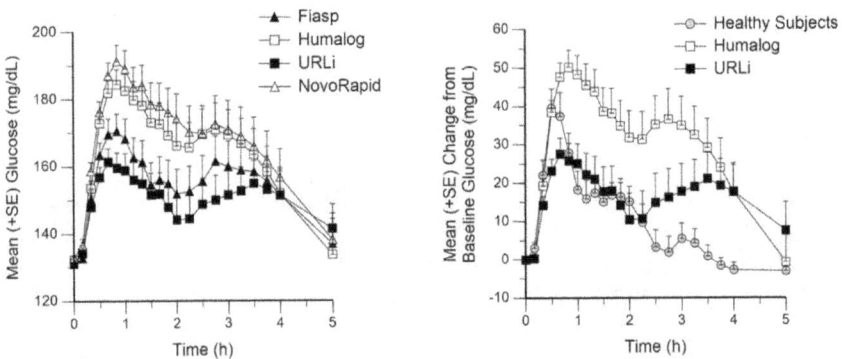

Figure 6.1—Comparison of the postprandial glucose lowering after a standardized test meal with a SC dose of URLi, Humalog, Fiasp, or NovoRapid (Left) and between Humalog, URLi, Healthy Subjects (Right). *Source:* Adapted with permission from Heise.[5]

SC, subcutaneous

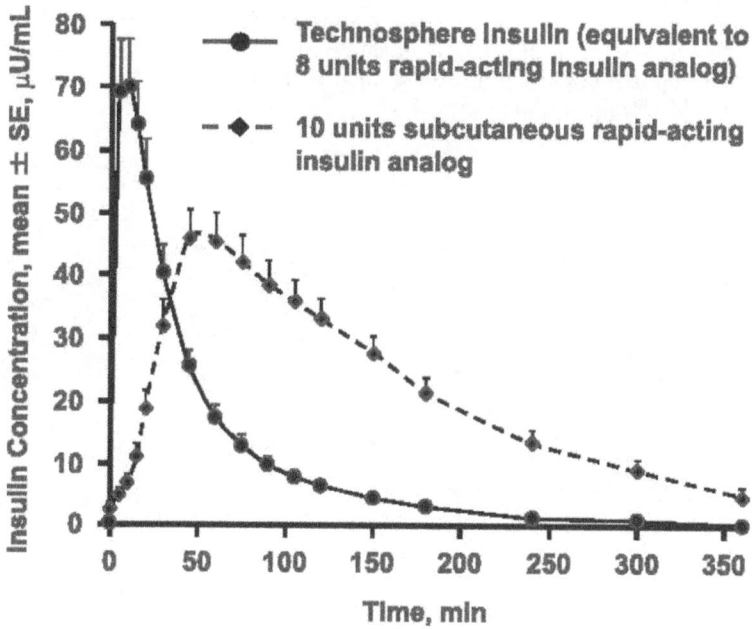

Figure 6.2—*Source*: Adapted from Leahy[13].

Rapid-Acting Insulin

Three genetically engineered insulin analogs designed to have a rapid onset and short duration of action when injected subcutaneously are currently available. Insulin lispro, [Lys(B28), Pro(B29)]-human insulin, contains an inversion of the amino acids at positions 28 and 29 of the B-chain. Insulin aspart, [Asp(B28)]-human insulin, contains a substitution of the proline at position 28 of the B-chain with aspartate.[14] Insulin glulisine contains a lysine at B3 replacing asparagine, and a glutamic acid at B29 replaces lysine.[15] These analogs have similar pharmacokinetic properties. They are sterile, aqueous, clear, and colorless, and they have a neutral pH. In contrast to native human insulin, the modifications in the insulin molecule inhibit its ability to self-aggregate into hexamers and dimers in solution. This enables insulin to be more rapidly absorbed from the subcutaneous tissue after injection.[15-24]

Short-Acting Insulin

Regular (soluble or unmodified) insulin has the most rapid onset and shortest duration of action of any native insulin preparation (i.e., human insulin that is not modified to change its pharmacokinetic properties) with an onset at 30–60 min, a peak effect 2–3 h after administration, and an effective duration of action of 3–6 h (Fig. 6.3). Because of interindividual variation, in some patients, an effect is evident for up to 8 h. Duration of action may be longer with large doses or when patients have insulin antibodies.[14,25]

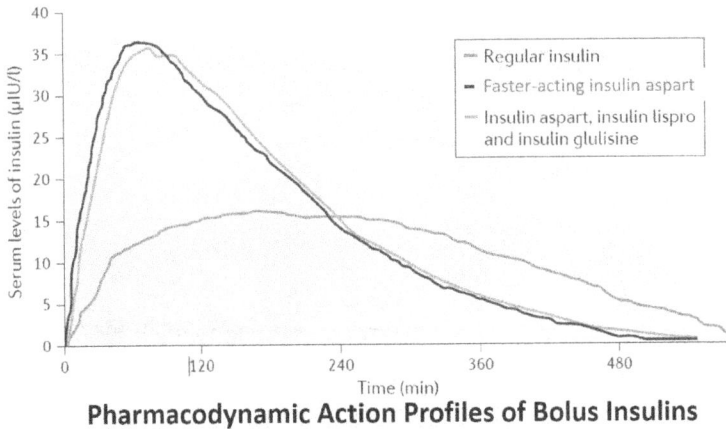

Pharmacodynamic Action Profiles of Bolus Insulins

Figure 6.3—*Source*: Adapted from Mathieu.[26]

Intermediate-Acting Insulin

NPH insulin, which is an intermediate-acting insulin, uses protamine to retard and extend insulin action. The addition of protamine creates an insulin suspension, and after injection, insulin is more slowly absorbed from the subcutaneous tissue. NPH insulin has an onset of action 2–4 h after injection, a peak effect 4–10 h after administration, and an effective duration of action of 10–16 h.[20,27–29]

Long-Acting Insulin

U-100 insulin glargine. U-100 insulin glargine is a genetically modified insulin analog (21^A-Gly-30^Ba-L-Arg-30^Bb-L-Arg-human insulin). The amino acid asparagine at position A21 is replaced by glycine, and two arginines are added to the C-terminus of the B-chain. The effect of these changes is to shift the isoelectric point, producing a solution that is completely soluble at pH 4. When injected into the subcutaneous tissue, which has a physiological pH of 7.4, the acidic solution is neutralized. This leads to the formation of microprecipitates, or stabilized aggregates, from which small amounts of insulin glargine are slowly released. Glargine is absorbed from abdominal subcutaneous injection sites at a relatively constant rate, with no prominent peak in serum insulin concentration for 24 h.[19,28,30–32]

Insulin detemir. Insulin detemir is a long-acting basal insulin analog with a duration of action up to 24 h. Insulin detemir differs from human insulin in that threonine has been omitted from position B30 and a C14 fatty acid chain has been attached to the amino acid at position B29. Insulin detemir is a clear, colorless, aqueous neutral sterile solution at pH 7.4. Its prolonged action is the result of slow systemic absorption of insulin detemir molecules from the injection site caused by strong self-association of the molecules and binding to albumin. Insulin detemir is more slowly distributed to peripheral target tissues because it is highly bound to albumin in the bloodstream. Compared with NPH, both insulin glargine and insulin detemir have less dose-to-dose variability in pharmacodynamics.[33-35]

Ultra-Long-Acting Insulin

Although long-acting insulin glargine is generally considered to have a 20–24-h duration of action, some individuals may not achieve full 24-h basal coverage. Some individuals may experience a rise in blood glucose toward the end of their dosing interval. For these individuals, it may be appropriate to consider an ultra-long-acting basal insulin with demonstrated longer duration of action.

U-300 insulin glargine. Insulin glargine is concentrated to contain 300 units insulin glargine per 1 mL. Before injection, U-300 insulin has pH 4, but upon injection the solution becomes neutralized, allowing a precipitate to form under the skin. From this precipitate, small amounts of insulin are released.[36] U-300 insulin glargine shows less fluctuation in its pharmacokinetic/pharmacodynamic profile as compared with U-100 insulin glargine, including decreased disparity in blood glucose values over the injection interval, and more stable activity on blood glucose control over a 24-h period with less hyperglycemic and/or hypoglycemic excursions, and it demonstrates decreased rise in blood glucose during the final 4 h of the injection interval. The concentrated version of insulin glargine has a duration of action lasting >24 h, and it offers greater flexibility in timing of daily injections as well as a decreased occurrence of nocturnal hypoglycemia as compared to U-100 insulin glargine, offering an improved safety profile.[37-39] The steady-state effectiveness is noted to be less than that of U-100 insulin glargine, however, and may require ~11–17% higher dose as compared with U-100 insulin glargine to maintain the same glucose-lowering effect.[36,39,40]

Insulin degludec. Insulin degludec (INN/USAN) is an ultra-long-acting insulin analog. It has one single amino acid deleted in comparison to human insulin and is conjugated to hexadecanedioic acid via γ-L-glutamyl spacer at the amino acid lysine at position B29. The addition of hexadecanedioic acid to lysine at the B29 position allows for the formation of multihexamers in subcutaneous tissue, or subcutaneous depot, that results in slow insulin release into the systemic circulation. The onset of action is 30–90 min, and its duration of action is up to 42 h. Because of its ultra-long action, it can be administered at any time of the day every day.[22,41,42]

Compared with U-100 insulin glargine, insulin degludec, similar to U-300 glargine, has lower incidence of nocturnal hypoglycemia in both type 2 diabetes (T2D) and T1D because of its low day-to-day variability.[41] It can be used at the same unit dose as the total daily long- or intermediate-acting insulin unit dose. Insulin degludec can also be mixed with short-acting insulin aspart.[26] See Fig. 6.4 for a graphic representation of intermediate, long, and ultra-long-acting insulin profiles.

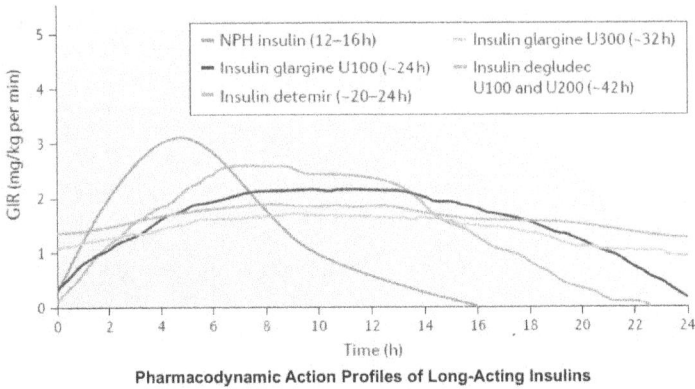

Pharmacodynamic Action Profiles of Long-Acting Insulins

Figure 6.4—*Source*: Reprinted with permission from Mathieu.[26]

Concentrated Formulations of Insulin

Several concentrated formulations of insulin have become available in recent years. Concentrated insulins help achieve smaller injection volumes, which may decrease pain and discomfort felt by the patient, enable larger dosages to be administered in one injection, and potentially limit the number of pen changes during the week/month.[43] Insulin in stable formulation in vials and pens is typically in hexameric form. In order to be absorbed into capillaries, insulin must dissociate from hexamers to dimers and monomers. This happens at lower concentrations of insulin, typically at the borders of the insulin depot when injected into subcutaneous tissue. Higher concentrations and lower volume of insulin injected result in fewer insulin molecules reaching the outside of the depot at one time, thus prolonging the absorption and creating more of a flattened, prolonged, and stable PK curve. Certain concentrated insulins (U-200 insulin lispro and U-200 insulin degludec) have been formulated to maintain bioequivalence to their nonconcentrated formulations.[43]

Concentrated insulin may be considered for patients with severe insulin resistance and those requiring large-volume injections.[44] These formulations have the same number of units in a smaller volume (e.g., U-200 has 200 units insulin in 1 mL, U-300 has 300 units in 1 mL) and are available in pens that display the number of units. The dose dialed on the pen by the patient is the dose dispensed by the device. It is important for clinicians to know how units are displayed for each product when prescribing insulin doses as well as the maximum number of units per injection (e.g., U-200 insulin degludec is dosed in 2-unit increments with a maximum delivery of 160 units per dose, whereas U-200 insulin lispro is dosed in 1-unit increments with a maximum delivery of 60 units per dose).

Concentrated U-200 faster-acting insulin lispro (Lyumjev U-200) is a concentrated formulation of U-100 faster-acting insulin lispro (Lyumjev U-100) that has pharmacokinetic parameters comparable to U-100 faster-acting insulin lispro. Equivalent dosages can be administered with half-volume injections.

Concentrated U-200 insulin lispro demonstrates pharmacokinetic parameters comparable to U-100 insulin lispro. Equivalent to the U-100 formulation, U-200 insulin lispro has the same change in its amino acid sequence (switch of lysine and proline), which contributes to a destabilization of hexamers in the injection depot, leading to a greater amount of insulin as dimers and monomers. To maintain bioequivalence, U-200 insulin lispro contains approximately doubled concentration of zinc ion, 0.046 mg/mL as compared to 0.0197 mg/mL in U-100 insulin lispro, facilitating similar hexamer formation and deceased rate of degradation. In addition, a change in buffering agent from phosphate to tromethamine helps to reduce phosphate salts (zinc phosphate) from precipitating from the higher concentration of zinc present in equivalent volume.[25,45] This version of insulin lispro allows for smaller injection volume while maintaining bioequivalence.[23,44]

Concentrated U-200 insulin degludec was developed to exhibit similar pharmacokinetic parameters as U-100 insulin degludec. U-200 insulin degludec forms the same long chains of hexamers, allowing for dissociation into dimers and monomers only at the end of these chains, extending its duration of action. It has demonstrated bioequivalence to U-100 insulin degludec and the two concentrations may be considered interchangeable.[42,44] This formulation of concentrated insulin degludec allows for equivalent dosing with decreased injection volume.

Concentrated U-300 insulin glargine demonstrates a more stable and truly peakless pharmacokinetic profile compared with U-100 insulin glargine over the course of dosing duration and causes less nocturnal hypoglycemia.[36-40] It is available currently in pen formulations of 1.5 mL (450 units) or 3 mL (900 units) per pen.[36]

Improvements with U-500 insulin have also been developed. U-500 insulin is indicated for patients who require >200 units of insulin per day. An insulin pen formulation and a U-500–specific insulin syringe with 5-unit increment markings are available. Patients and clinicians have three options to administer U-500 insulin, including syringe and vial, insulin pen, or insulin pump. It is a high-risk medication and patients and clinicians need extensive education to avoid dosing errors. The U-500 insulin pen is dosed in 5-unit increments providing patients with the actual dose of insulin to be injected up to a maximum of 300 units per injection. For patients who require vial and syringe, the U-500 insulin syringe was created to reduce dosing errors and the need for providers to calculate syringe units for patients. The U-500 insulin syringe allows patients to inject doses in 5-unit increments up to a maximum of 250 units per injection. It is imperative for patients to alert healthcare providers if they are using the U-500 insulin pen, U-500 insulin syringe, U-100 insulin syringe, or a tuberculin syringe to administer U-500 insulin to avoid dosing errors.[46-49]

Insulin Mixtures

There are commercially prepared, stable mixtures of regular and NPH insulins, insulin lispro protamine suspension (NPL) and insulin lispro, and insulin aspart protamine suspension (NPA) and insulin aspart. These mixtures contain either 70% NPH and 30% regular insulin, or 50% NPL and 50% insulin lispro (called "50/50"), or 75% NPL and 25% insulin lispro (called "75/25"), or 70% NPA and 30% insulin aspart (called "70/30"). These premixed insulins may be helpful in patients who are blind or elderly, patients with cognitive impairment, or other patients who have difficulty using complex insulin regimens. These mixtures limit flexible dosing, however, and necessitate that the patient be on a fixed meal plan, which incorporates planned snacking in the midmorning after breakfast and potentially between dinnertime and bedtime to avoid hypoglycemia.[50-54]

Another approved mixture with ultra-long-acting insulin degludec and insulin aspart consists of 70% insulin degludec and 30% insulin aspart. This insulin formulation can be given once a day using a dose corresponding to 70% of total daily dose, with the remaining 30% split and given as insulin aspart at the other meals.[22,55]

Follow-on Biologic Insulins

Follow-on biologic insulins, "biosimilars," are created to be highly similar to the reference insulin product. They are analogous to generic versions of small-molecule drugs. Manufacturers of follow-on biologic insulins use techniques that are similar but not identical to those used by the reference product's manufacturer. They may differ slightly in their molecular characteristics, clinical profiles, and immunogenicity. Currently available biosimilars include insulin glargine and insulin lispro. They are dosed using a 1:1 ratio to their reference products; however, when switching to a biosimilar, dose adjustments may be necessary based on individual patient requirements. With continued development of follow-on biologic insulin options, clinicians and patients may benefit from an increase in access to modern insulin therapy and an overall reduction of medical costs.[56-61]

STABILITY OF INSULINS

Insulin is stable for long periods of time when refrigerated; therefore, it should be stored in a refrigerator (this includes insulin human inhalation powder). Injectable insulin is generally stable at room temperature for 28 days and does not need to be stored in the refrigerator after the bottle or pen is opened, as long as it is used within this time frame. Sealed unopened blister cards and strips of insulin human inhalation powder are stable at room temperature for up to 10 days, whereas opened strips should be used within 3 days. Insulin should not be exposed to extreme temperatures, such as direct sunlight, excessive heat, or freezing temperatures (e.g., in a car, near a window, or by a heating or air conditioning vent).[62]

Regular insulin and the synthetic insulin analogs (lispro, aspart, glulisine, detemir, glargine, and degludec) are all in solution. All other insulin preparations except insulin human inhalation powder are in suspension. Vials containing NPH, NPL, and NPA insulin suspensions must be gently rolled at least 10 times (it has been recommended that pens containing NPH insulin be rolled and tipped

20 times) to ensure uniform suspension before insulin is withdrawn from the vial or injected using a pen.

On mixing insulins, physiochemical changes may occur (either immediately or over time). As a result, the physiological response to the insulin mixture may differ from that of the insulins injected separately. Mixtures of two types of insulin vary in stability. Regular, lispro, aspart, glulisine, and NPH-type insulins are freely miscible in all proportions. These insulins may be mixed in the same syringe and their action profiles may be maintained. A decrease in the absorption rate (but not total bioavailability) is seen when insulin lispro, aspart, or glulisine are mixed with NPH insulin. Most or all of the rapid action of regular insulin or the rapid-acting analogs is retained if mixing is done in a syringe immediately before injection. Ultra-rapid insulin analogs should not be mixed with other insulins. The acidic nature of insulin glargine precludes its mixture with other insulins. Insulin detemir should not be mixed with any other insulins because it can substantially reduce their absorption profile.Insulin degludec should not be mixed with any other insulins, unless in the U.S. Food and Drug Administration (FDA) approved combination pen with insulin aspart.[32,35,36,42,55]

INSULIN ABSORPTION

Many factors influence insulin absorption and alter insulin availability. Intra-individual variation in insulin absorption from day to day can vary by as much as 25%, and between patients up to 50%. The long-acting insulin analogs degludec, glargine, and detemir have less dose-to-dose variability in pharmacodynamics than intermediate-acting insulin NPH. In general, as the dose is increased, the absorption of subcutaneously injected insulin becomes more prolonged.[43,62]

Injection Site

Insulin absorption differs across injection sites, especially for ultra-rapid, rapid-acting, and short-acting insulins (faster-acting aspart, faster-acting lispro, aspart, lispro, glulisine, and regular). Absorption is most rapid from the abdomen, followed by the arm, buttocks, and thigh. These differences are likely the result of variation in subcutaneous blood flow. The variation is great enough that random rotation of preprandial or correctional insulin injection sites should be avoided, if possible. Patients should rotate injection sites within regions, rather than between regions, for any given injection to decrease day-to-day variability. Because insulin absorption is most rapid in the abdomen (in the absence of exercise), it may be the preferred site for preprandial injections. Some patients use the abdomen for all preprandial injections, whereas others use the abdomen for the prebreakfast injection and other regions for prelunch or predinner injections.[31,62]

Timing of Premeal Injections

Timing of preprandial insulin injections is crucial to matching insulin action with carbohydrate absorption. Human insulin inhalation powder should be inhaled immediately prior to the meal. Fiasp has an onset of action ~5 min sooner than conventional rapid-acting aspart and may be injected closer to the onset of a meal.[1] Insulin lispro, glulisine, and aspart have a rapid onset of action and generally should be given ~15 min before starting to eat a meal. Subcutaneous regular insulin should be injected at least 20–30 min before eating a meal.

With more rapidly absorbed high glycemic index carbohydrate meals, it is sometimes necessary to bolus even earlier to provide appropriate coverage for the meal. Conversely, early administration of insulin before meals containing slowly digested lower glycemic index carbohydrates can result in early postprandial hypoglycemia. In these situations, insulin is best given immediately before the meal. In practice, review of continuous glucose monitoring (CGM) tracings can be informative in defining optimal bolus timing for specific meals. The timing of injections also should be altered depending on premeal glycemia. When blood glucose levels are above a patient's target range, the interval between insulin administration and meal consumption should be increased to permit the insulin to lower blood glucose toward the target range. For example, when the premeal glucose is above target, rapid-acting insulin can be given 15–30 min and regular insulin 30–60 min before the meal. If premeal blood glucose levels are below a patient's target range, regular insulin should be injected immediately before meal consumption, while rapid-acting insulin analog administration should be delayed until after the blood glucose level has been restored to normal. In certain circumstances (if the ability of the patient to consume the meal is uncertain), it is prudent to wait until immediately after completing the meal to administer rapid-acting insulin. The presence of gastroparesis diabeticorum may significantly delay carbohydrate absorption. In these patients, postmeal insulin administration or the use of regular insulin, which has a longer onset of action, may be advantageous.[15,17,18,63,64]

Factors Influencing Insulin Absorption

Physical exercise increases blood flow to an exercising body part and accelerates absorption of insulin from that region. Sporadic exercise may induce variability in insulin absorption. The patient should avoid injections in a body region that will be exercised while that injection is being absorbed. For example, if the patient intends to jog shortly after an injection, he or she should avoid giving that injection into the thigh. When exercise is contemplated, the patient might use the abdomen preferentially, because this region is the least likely to have significant increases in absorption (unless sit-ups are planned). Other factors influencing absorption of regular insulin are ambient temperature (e.g., a hot bath or sauna), smoking, and local massage of the injection site.

Thin patients with little subcutaneous tissue face an increased risk of intramuscular rather than subcutaneous injection with longer needle lengths, which leads to more rapid absorption of any given insulin preparation. This risk can be averted by using short needles.[65] Needles of 4, 5, and 6 mm may be used by any adult patient, including patients who are obese, and do not generally require lifting of the skinfold.[62] Also, the interval between injection of preprandial insulin and meal consumption may need to be shortened.

Any patient injecting insulin should be monitored for development of insulin lipohypertrophy or lipoatrophy at sites of injection. Injection into these areas may result in delayed or sporadic absorption of insulin and should be avoided.

MULTICOMPONENT INSULIN REGIMENS: GENERAL POINTS

There are two components of physiological insulin secretion: continuous basal insulin secretion and incremental prandial insulin secretion (see Fig. 6.5). Basal insulin secretion restrains hepatic glucose production, keeping it in equilibrium with basal glucose use by the brain and other tissues that are obligate glucose consumers. After meals, prandial insulin secretion stimulates glucose use and storage while inhibiting hepatic glucose output, thereby limiting the meal-related glucose excursion. The most flexible regimens used for intensive diabetes management are those that[66]

- emphasize the need for preprandial insulin before each meal, separate from basal insulin;
- allow liberal food choices in terms of size, timing, and potential omission of meals while still balancing food intake with activity and insulin dosage; and
- include frequent monitoring of therapy to promote a more normal lifestyle.[67]

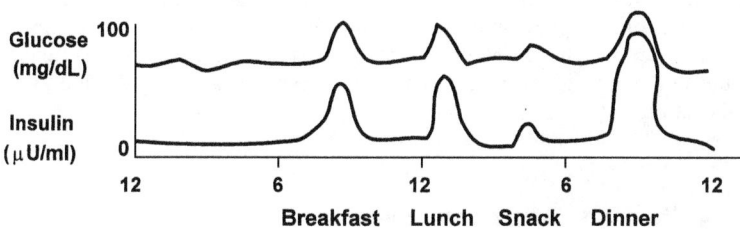

Figure 6.5—Schematic representation of 24-h plasma glucose and insulin profiles in a hypothetical individual without diabetes.

Instrumental to the overall plan is frequent monitoring of glucose data, best achieved via the incorporation of CGM or self-monitoring of blood glucose via fingerstick (SMBG) multiple times daily. The patient takes action based on the SMBG or CGM results, which are used to help make appropriate changes in insulin dosage and timing, carbohydrate intake, and physical activity. The changes are made according to a predetermined plan agreed upon by the healthcare team and the patient.[20,30]

Prandial Insulin Therapy

Prandial incremental insulin secretion is best replicated by giving preprandial ultra-rapid-acting insulin (insulin human inhalation powder, faster-acting insulin aspart, faster-acting insulin lispro) or a rapid-acting insulin analog (lispro, aspart, or glulisine) before each meal by inhalation, syringe, pen, or pump. Each prepran-dial insulin dose is adjusted individually to provide an amount of insulin appropriate to the current and anticipated blood glucose level (if CGM is being used) and the meal. If exercise is planned after the meal, insulin doses may need to be reduced. Dietary fat and protein can affect mealtime insulin requirements (see Chapter 9, Nutrition Management), and insulin doses may need to be adjusted.[30,63,64]

Basal Insulin Therapy

Basal insulin is given as

- one or two daily injections of long-acting insulin (U-100 glargine or detemir) or a single injection of ultra-long-acting insulin (degludec, U-200 degludec, or U-300 glargine),
- intermediate-acting insulin (NPH) at bedtime and in the morning, or
- the basal component of a continuous subcutaneous insulin infusion (CSII) program.

SPECIFIC FLEXIBLE MULTICOMPONENT INSULIN REGIMENS

Premeal Rapid- and Basal Long-Acting Insulins

A premeal program uses preprandial insulin injections of either ultra-rapid (insulin human inhalation powder, faster-acting aspart, faster-acting lispro) or rapid-acting insulin (lispro, aspart, or glulisine) and long-acting degludec, glargine, or detemir insulin to provide basal insulin (see Figs. 6.6 and 6.7). If given twice a day, insulin detemir is a relatively peakless insulin. Glargine is also peakless in most patients when given once a day, and it reaches a steady state 3–5 h after administration.[34,63]

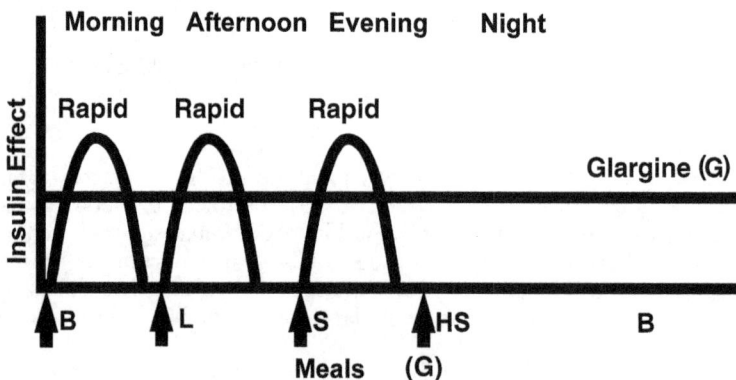

Figure 6.6—Schematic representation of idealized insulin effect provided by multiple-dose regimen providing basal long-acting insulin glargine (G) and preprandial injections of rapid-acting insulin. B, breakfast; L, lunch; S, dinner; HS, bedtime. Arrows indicate time of insulin injection. Although frequently given at HS, the basal insulin may be given at other times of the day and may be required twice a day.

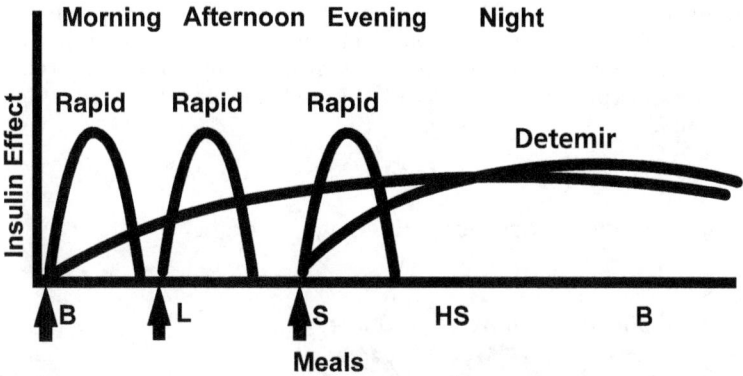

Figure 6.7—Schematic representation of idealized insulin effect provided by multiple-dose regimen providing basal long-acting insulin detemir and preprandial injections of rapid-acting insulin. B, breakfast; L, lunch; S, dinner; HS, bedtime. Arrows indicate time of insulin injection. Although frequently given at HS, insulin detemir is often injected twice a day.

Insulin degludec is relatively peakless after injection and has a sustained duration of action of >42 h. Because it lasts >24 h, the low day-to-day variation in its glucose-lowering effect allows patients who forget a dose, or who for other reasons cannot administer their scheduled dose, greater flexibility in dosing time.

U-100 insulin glargine has a broad peak 15–18 h after injection and a sustained action of 20–24 h. It is sufficiently peakless to provide adequate daily basal insulin. If given with dinner, the waning effect after 18–20 h may result in late-afternoon hyperglycemia; therefore, bedtime administration may provide better coverage.[39]

Insulin detemir has a broad peak 6–8 h after injection and, when given twice a day, may have sustained action up to 24 h.[35] In most patients, twice-daily detemir at steady state has such a sufficiently blunted peak that it behaves like a peakless basal insulin. As a consequence of the waning insulin effect after 20–24 h, if insulin detemir is administered as a single morning dose, glucose levels may increase before the next injection. Thus, it is best to divide detemir insulin into two doses.[33] In practice, detemir can optimize glucose control in individuals who have different day versus night basal requirements and in those who want the flexibility to adjust basal insulin (analogous to the use of the pump temporary basal feature to compensate for increased activity).

Premeal Rapid- and Basal Intermediate-Acting Insulins

This older premeal regimen, which is less commonly prescribed, uses three preprandial insulin injections (lispro, glulisine, or aspart) and intermediate-acting insulin (NPH) given at bedtime to provide overnight basal insulin with peak serum insulin levels before breakfast (a time of a relative increase in insulin requirements because of insulin resistance known as the "dawn phenomenon"; see Fig. 6.8). Bedtime administration of intermediate-acting insulin also reduces the risk of nocturnal hypoglycemia. A small morning dose of intermediate-acting insulin (perhaps 20–30% of the bedtime dose) provides daytime basal insulin.[63]

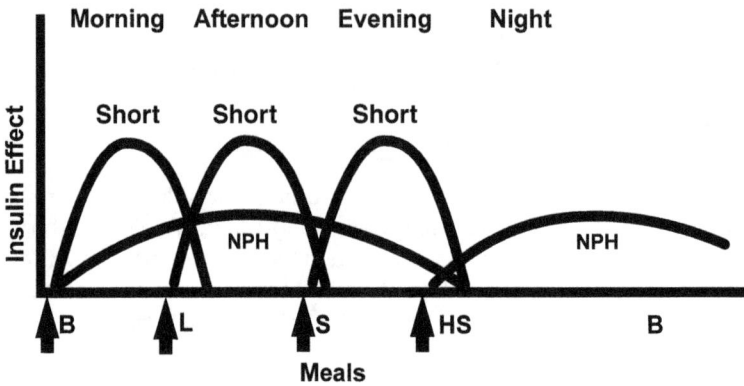

(a)

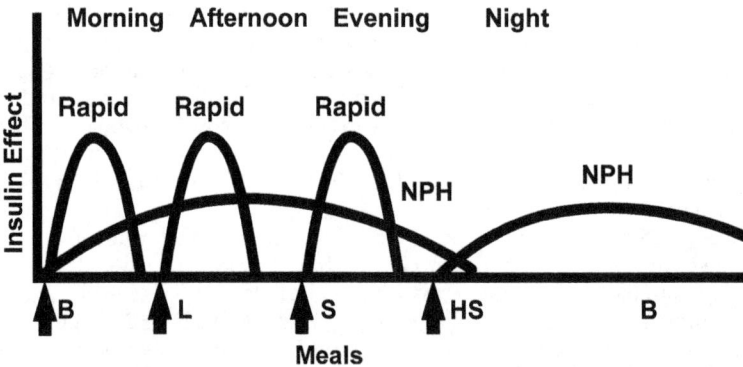

(b)

Figure 6.8—Schematic representation of idealized insulin effect provided by multiple-dose regimen providing basal intermediate-acting insulin at bedtime and before breakfast and preprandial injections of short- (a) or rapid- (b) acting insulin. B, breakfast; L, lunch; S, dinner; HS, bedtime. Arrows indicate time of insulin injection.

The basal-bolus regimen is popular for a variety of reasons. It offers flexibility in meal size and timing if the dose is adjusted (if a fixed dose is taken, the same amount of carbohydrates should be consumed). This regimen is straightforward and easy to understand and implement, because each meal and each period of the day has a well-defined insulin component providing primary insulin action.

Continuous Subcutaneous Insulin Infusion

The most accurate and convenient way to mimic normal insulin secretion is to use CSII, also referred to as insulin pump therapy (see Fig. 6.9). The pump continually delivers ultra-rapid-acting (faster-acting aspart) or rapid-acting insulin analog (lispro, aspart, glulisine), thus replicating basal insulin secretion. Moreover, to optimize glycemia, the basal rate may be adjusted frequently in a hybrid closed-loop system that uses an algorithm to automate insulin delivery based on real-time CGM glucose inputs. A pump can also be programmed to vary the rate of basal insulin delivery at times of diurnal variation in insulin sensitivity that adversely effect glycemic control. Thus, the basal infusion rate may be decreased overnight to avert nocturnal hypoglycemia or may be increased to counteract the dawn phenomenon, which often results in hyperglycemia on waking. Temporary basal rates may be used and different patterns may be established, corresponding to the needs of shift workers or people with differing amounts of physical activity on given days. For more on CSII, see Chapter 7.

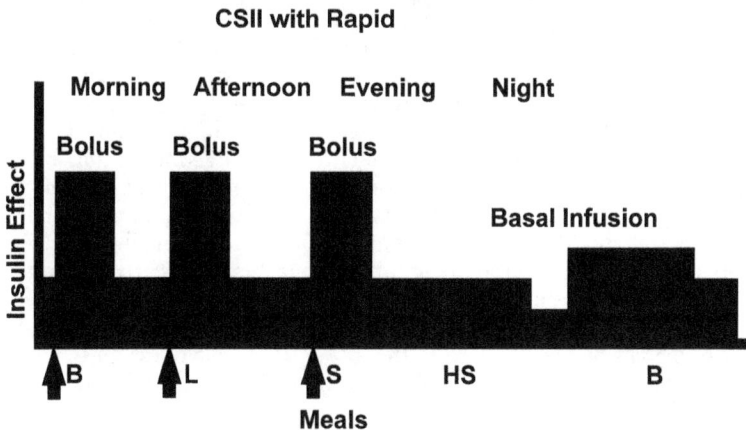

Figure 6.9—Schematic representation of idealized insulin effect provided by CSII of rapid-acting insulin. B, breakfast; L, lunch; S, dinner; HS, bedtime. Arrows indicate time of insulin injection.

TYPE 1 DIABETES

Individuals living with T1D require insulin regimens with multiple components that mimic physiological insulin secretion—providing basal and prandial insulin with each meal. Mimicking normal physiological insulin necessitates delivery of basal insulin between meals and overnight. Basal insulin should be combined with periodic boluses of prandial insulin that aim to coincide with the rise in glucose that accompanies food ingestion. The final component of what is frequently called "basal-bolus-correctional" insulin programs is the periodic administration of rapid-acting insulin boluses to restore euglycemia when an individual's blood glucose is above target range. These correction boluses may be added to preprandial boluses if the patient plans to eat at the time of the bolus or can be delivered as standalone boluses to "correct" hyperglycemic excursions.

In typical patients with T1D who are within 20% of their ideal body weight, in the absence of an intercurrent infection or other cause of metabolic instability or insulin resistance, the total daily insulin dose required for glycemic control is usually 0.3–1.0 unit/kg/day. The dose is lower during the remission or honeymoon period early in the course of the disease (e.g., 0.2–0.6 unit/kg/day). Moreover, during the remission or honeymoon period, as a result of some continuing endogenous insulin secretion, it may be relatively easy to achieve near-normal glycemic control with virtually any insulin program.[31]

During intercurrent illness, puberty, and pregnancy, the insulin requirements may increase markedly (even doubling). Doses (in units per kilogram) progressively increase during pregnancy, typically starting in the mid second trimester. Because the patient's weight also increases, the total dose may even triple, although this is far more common in women with T2D and gestational diabetes than in T1D. Insulin requirements typically increase throughout puberty and may reach 1.3–1.5 units/kg/day during the adolescent growth spurt.[68]

NPH at breakfast time is sometimes used in young children who attend school where there is no school nurse to give lunchtime rapid-acting insulin. The NPH at breakfast provides insulin coverage for the morning snack and lunch at school.

In general, ~40–50% of the total daily insulin dose is used to provide basal insulin. The remainder is divided among the meals, traditionally primarily proportionate to the carbohydrate content of the meals. As a starting point, when optimizing prandial insulin dosing, bolus doses are calculated based on the number of grams of carbohydrate consumed. Ultimately, the goal is for the patient to be able to match the meal boluses to the intake of carbohydrate at each meal and snack with an individualized ratio of 1 unit of insulin per specific amount of carbohydrate. This is called the insulin-to-carbohydrate ratio. In practice, it is useful to ask the patient to follow a prescribed meal plan based on the patient's usual dietary intake to establish the patient's insulin-to-carbohydrate ratio. In children, the ratio of insulin to carbohydrate depends on age, body size, pubertal status, and activity level, with a range of 0.3–1.0 unit for every 10 g of carbohydrate consumed. The insulin-to-carbohydrate ratio should be individualized through the use of dietary intake records and review of blood glucose responses.

Breakfast generally requires a slightly larger amount of insulin per gram of carbohydrate and there may be individual reasons for differences at other times of day as well. Alternatively, a constant carbohydrate diet can be prescribed with a fixed insulin dose based on the prescribed carbohydrate content (see Chapter 9). Some patients may desire or require a dose of rapid-acting insulin to cover a bedtime snack. It is important to recognize that food macronutrient groups other than carbohydrates (fats, proteins) and the type of carbohydrates consumed (e.g., white rice versus steel-cut oats) in addition to the mix of macronutrients consumed at each individual meal, all play a role in postprandial glucose excursions. Advanced CSII prandial insulin delivery strategies, including extended boluses, are often useful to address the delayed postprandial glycemic excursions that occur after high-fat or high-protein meals. More detail is included in Chapter 7 and Chapter 9. Carbohydrate counting should be regarded as a useful, although imperfect, basis for determining prandial insulin delivery. Our ultimate goal should be to encourage patients to learn how to carefully match their individual and unique meal choices with appropriate insulin delivery strategies that are likely to vary from meal to meal. Future research into personalized decision support tools based on individualized insulin, CGM, and activity data will further refine our ability to individualize prandial insulin doses.

TYPE 2 DIABETES

T2D is a progressive disease and many patients eventually require insulin therapy. Insulin should always be considered in individuals with severe hyperglycemia, especially if catabolic features (weight loss, hypertriglyceridemia, ketosis) are present, or when patients are not meeting glycemic goals despite multiple noninsulin glucose-lowering therapies. Basal insulin is often the most convenient insulin to initiate when insulin therapy is considered and is often added to other noninsulin agents. Starting doses can be estimated based on body weight, starting at 0.1–0.2 unit/kg/day. Clinicians should be aware of the potential for over-basalization with insulin therapy. Clinical signs that may prompt evaluation include basal dose more than ~0.5 unit/kg/day, high bedtime–morning glucose differential (>50 mg/dL), hypoglycemia, and high variability. If the A1C remains above target after initiation of basal insulin, addition of prandial insulin with one or more meals may be considered. Typically this dose is either 10% of the basal insulin dose or the common practice of 4 units, administered before the largest meal or the meal resulting in the greatest postprandial glucose excursion. If the A1C remains elevated, further adjustments and intensification will be required.[67]

INSULIN ADJUSTMENTS

Patients are provided with an action plan to alter their therapy to achieve individual, defined blood glucose targets before and after meals, at bedtime, and overnight. Actions may include changing the timing of insulin injections in relation to meals, changing the amount or content of food to be consumed, or altering insulin doses.

ACUTE ADJUSTMENTS

Acute adjustments may include changes in food intake and in timing of insulin administration as well as changes in insulin dosage. In practice, most patients find adjustments in the insulin dose to be the most convenient adjustment to make. For severely low blood glucose values, however, additional carbohydrate is urgently needed, and for exceptionally high blood glucose values, a delay in the meal after the insulin dose may be needed. Many experts avoid the term "sliding scale," because the traditional sliding scale did not recognize ongoing (basal and prandial) insulin requirements and would prescribe no insulin when the blood glucose level was in the target range.

Acute adjustments are intended to correct momentary deviations of blood glucose outside the target range and frequently are referred to as "correction doses." The correction may be used when the person experiences a variation in activity, intercurrent illness, or other stress or needs to correct variations in glycemia. The correction dose is in addition to the usual prandial and basal doses.

Corrections actually may be decrements (negative corrections, e.g., lowering of preprandial insulin in anticipation of postprandial exercise or in the face of prevailing blood glucose levels lower than the preprandial target). For patients on a constant carbohydrate diet, corrections (positive or negative) may be given for a larger or smaller carbohydrate meal.[69]

Preprandial corrections provide an action plan for the patient guided by CGM or SMBG determinations and daily records. Calculations for corrective insulin doses are given in Chapter 7. One method of calculating the "correction factor" (i.e., the amount of additional insulin needed with a meal to restore the blood glucose to the target level) is to use the "rule of 1,500 or 1,800." To calculate, 1,500 or 1,800 is divided by the total daily dose of insulin to estimate the effect of rapid-acting insulin on the blood glucose level. In a patient with a blood glucose level of 250 mg/dL and an insulin sensitivity (or correction) factor of 1 unit per 50 mg/dL, the correction dose would be 3 units of rapid-acting insulin for a target glucose of 100 mg/dL. Obese patients with T2D typically are insulin resistant and require a higher correction dose, as calculated by the previous formula.

Dosing decision-making will depend on the answers to several questions that the patient asks at the time of any premeal insulin injection:

- What is my blood glucose now?
- What do I plan to eat now (i.e., how much carbohydrate and fat will I consume)?
- Do I plan to have an alcoholic beverage with the meal?
- What do I plan to do after eating (i.e., usual activity, increased activity, or decreased activity)?
- What did I do in the past hour (i.e., usual activity, increased activity, or decreased activity)?
- What has happened under these circumstances previously?

The answers to these questions dictate the treatment response and become sensible routine decisions. The usual intervention is an adjustment in the insulin dose, but alterations in food intake (altering the amount or content of food), activity, and timing of injections in relation to meals also may be used.

PATTERN ADJUSTMENTS

Pattern analysis allows for adjustment in the insulin dose when the blood glucose is consistently above or below the target range at a particular time of day. When a pattern is identified, action should be taken to correct the high or low blood glucose at that time of day (see Table 6.2). The insulin dose (of the relevant insulin component most likely responsible) must be either increased or decreased to correct the pattern of glycemia outside the target range. Pattern analysis with insulin dose adjustments allows prospective changes to be made based on analysis of retrospective data. Pattern analysis can be especially effective when CGM is used, either retrospectively to evaluate diurnal changes in glucose levels, or prospectively to aid the patient to make dose adjustments. These adjustments do not depend on the blood glucose at the moment when they are implemented. Instead, they anticipate the insulin need for the future.

Table 6.2—Glucose Pattern Analysis Plan

This plan assumes that the preprandial and bedtime blood glucose target is 80–130 mg/dL. Plans should be individualized for each patient.

Insulin assumptions

- Basal insulin (bedtime NPH, detemir, glargine, degludec) is the major insulin acting overnight. Its effect is reflected in the results of blood glucose measurements during the middle of the night and on arising the next morning.
- Basal insulin (morning NPH, detemir, glargine, degludec) is the insulin acting and affecting glucose levels when meals are skipped and in the later morning and later afternoon (i.e., >4 h after the premeal insulin dose).
- Prebreakfast ultra-rapid-acting (faster-acting aspart, faster-acting lispro, insulin human inhalation powder) or rapid-acting insulin (lispro, aspart, glulisine) have major action after breakfast. The effect is primarily reflected in the results of blood glucose measurements 2–3 h after breakfast.
- Prelunch ultra-rapid-acting (faster-acting aspart, faster-acting lispro, insulin human inhalation powder) or rapid-acting insulin (lispro, aspart, glulisine) have major action after lunch. The effect is primarily reflected in the results of blood glucose measurements 2–3 h after lunch.
- Predinner ultra-rapid-acting (faster-acting aspart, faster-acting lispro, insulin human inhalation powder) or rapid-acting insulin (lispro, aspart, glulisine) have major action between dinner and bedtime. The effect is primarily reflected in the results of blood glucose tests 2–3 h after dinner.

If postprandial testing is not being performed, a pattern of rising of premeal and bedtime BG throughout the day with overnight correction may reflect excessive basal insulin relative to prandial insulin, with insufficiency of prandial dosing. This pattern often can be inferred without having many results of 2–3 h postprandial testing.[34,69]

INJECTION DEVICES

Making insulin injections easier and more comfortable enables patients to comply with a treatment plan.[70] In particular, patients may be more willing to initiate intensive diabetes management if a multiple daily insulin injection regimen is made more convenient.[71] Examples of injection devices include insulin pens and an injection port.[30,61]

Insulin pens are especially useful in intensive insulin therapy. Insulin cartridges containing units of regular, lispro, aspart, glulisine, NPH, 75/25, 50/50, or 70/30 insulin are placed in a pen-like device. Prefilled disposable pens are also available. Disposable needles (variable lengths, 4–12.7 mm) are attached to the end of the insulin pen. The desired dose is administered by turning a dial selector, plunging the needle into the subcutaneous tissue, and pushing a button at the end of the insulin pen to inject the insulin. Insulin pens are convenient to carry in a pocket, purse, backpack, or briefcase and make insulin injections easy to administer away from home. They eliminate the need to draw up insulin frequently throughout the day.

An injection port includes small needles or Teflon catheters with an external port that can be inserted into subcutaneous tissue of the abdomen or other sites and remain in place for several days. Injections can be given through the catheter instead of through the skin, thus reducing the number of needle punctures.

CONCLUSION

Intensive diabetes management involves flexible multicomponent insulin regimens tailored to the lifestyle of the patient.[20,70] These regimens consist of basal insulin and preprandial insulin, using separate insulin components for different times of the day. Therapy is guided by frequent SMBG and/or CGM. Patients follow action plans that guide them in daily self-management—altering insulin doses and timing, food intake, or activity—to achieve the selected target level of glycemia. Patient education, collaboration, and motivation are critical to successful program implementation.

REFERENCES

1. Fiasp [package insert]. Bagsvaerd, Denmark, Novo Nordisk A/S, 2019

2. Mathieu C. Developments in the management of type 1 and type 2 diabetes. *Eur Endocrinol* 2018;14(2):13–14

3. Heise T, Pieber TR, Kanne T, et al. A pooled analysis of clinical pharmacology trials investigating the pharmacokinetic and pharmacodynamics characteristics of fast-acting insulin aspart in adults with type 1 diabetes. *Clin Pharmacokinet* 2017;56(5):551–559

4. Shiramoto M, Nasu R, Oura T, et al. Ultra-rapid lispro results in accelerated insulin lispro absorption and fast early insulin action in comparison with Humalog® in Japanese patients with type 1 diabetes. *J Diabetes Investig* 2020;11(3):672–680

5. Heise T, Linnebjerg H, Cao D, et al. 1112-P: ultra rapid lispro (URLi) lowers postprandial glucose (PPG) and more closely matches normal physiological glucose response compared with other rapid insulin analogs. *Diabetes* 2019;68(Suppl. 1)

6. Klaff L, Cao D, Dellva MA, et al. Ultra rapid lispro improves postprandial glucose control compared with lispro in patients with type 1 diabetes: results from the 26-week PRONTO-T1D Study. *Diabetes Obes Metab* 2020;22(10): 1799–1807

7. Mathieu C, Bode BW, Franek E, et al. Efficacy and safety of fast-acting insulin aspart in comparison with insulin aspart in type 1 diabetes (onset 1): a 52-week, randomized, treat-to-target, phase III trial. *Diabetes Obes Metab* 2018;20:1148–1155

8. Russell-Jones D, Heller SR, Buchs S, et al. Projected long-term outcomes in patients with type 1 diabetes treated with fast-acting insulin vs conventional insulin aspart in the UK setting. *Diabetes Obes Metab* 2017;19:1773–1780

9. Russell-Jones D, Bode BW, De Block C, et al. Fast-acting insulin aspart improves glycemic control in basal-bolus treatment for type 1 diabetes: results of a 26-week multicenter, active-controlled, treat-to-target, randomized, parallel-group trial (onset 1). *Diabetes Care* 2017;40:943–950

10. Bode BW, McGill JB, Lorder DL, et al. Inhaled Technosphere insulin compared with injected prandial insulin in type 1 diabetes: a randomized 24-week trial. *Diabetes Care* 2015;38:2266–2273

11. Afrezza [package insert]. Danbury, CT, MannKind Corp., 2014

12. Fala L. Afrezza (insulin human) inhalation powder approved for the treatment of patients with type 1 diabetes or type 2 diabetes. *Am Health Drug Benefits* 2015;8:40–43

13. Leahy J. Technosphere inhaled insulin: is faster better? *Diabetes Care* 2015;38(12):2282–2284

14. Vajo Z, Duckworth WC. Genetically engineered insulin analogs: diabetes in the new millennium. *Pharmacol Rev* 2000;52:1–9

15. Hoogma RPLM, Schumicki D. Safety of insulin glulisine when given by continuous subcutaneous infusion using an external pump in patients with type 1 diabetes. *Horm Metab Res* 2006;38:429–433

16. Heise T, Heinemann L. Rapid and long-acting analogs as an approach to improve insulin therapy: an evidence-based medicine assessment. *Curr Pharm Des* 2001;7:1303–1325

17. Apidra [package insert]. Bridgewater, NJ, Sanofi-Aventis U.S. LLC, 2008

18. Becker RHA. Insulin glulisine complementing basal insulins: a review of structure and activity. *Diabetes Technol Therap* 2007;9(1):109–121

19. Grey M, Boland EA, Tamborlane WV. Use of lispro insulin and quality of life in adolescents on intensive therapy. *Diabetes Educ* 1999;25:934–941

20. Colombel A, Murat A, Krempf M, et al. Improvement of blood glucose control in type 1 diabetic patients treated with lispro and multiple NPH injections. *Diabetic Med* 1999;16:319–324

21. Tsui E, Barnie A, Ross S, et al. Intensive insulin therapy with insulin lispro: a randomized trial of continuous subcutaneous insulin infusion versus multiple daily insulin injection. *Diabetes Care* 2001;24:1722–1727

22. Hirsch IB, Bode B, Courreges JP, et al. Insulin degludec/insulin aspart administered once daily at any meal, with insulin aspart at other meals versus a standard basal-bolus regimen in patients with type 1 diabetes: a 26-week, phase 3, randomized, open-label, treat-to-target trial. *Diabetes Care* 2012;35(11):2174–2181

23. Humalog [package insert]. Indianapolis, IN, Lilly USA, LLC, 2020

24. Novolog [package insert]. Plainsboro, NJ, Novo Nordisk Inc., 2019

25. Humulin-R [package insert]. Indianapolis, IN, Lilly USA, LLC, 2019

26. Mathieu C, Gillard P, Benhalima K. Insulin analogues in type 1 diabetes mellitus: getting better all the time. *Nat Rev Endocrinol* 2017;13(7):385–399

27. Ratner RE, Hirsch IB, Neifing JL, et al. Less hypoglycemia with insulin glargine in intensive insulin therapy for type 1 diabetes. U.S. Study Group of Insulin Glargine in Type 1 Diabetes. *Diabetes Care* 2000;23:639–643

28. Rosenstock J, Park G, Zimmerman J, U.S. Insulin Glargine (HOE 901) Type 1 Diabetes Investigator Group. Basal insulin glargine (HOE 901) versus NPH insulin in patients with type 1 diabetes on multiple daily insulin regimens. *Diabetes Care* 2000;23:1127–1142

29. Humulin-N [package insert]. Indianapolis, IN, Lilly USA, LLC, 2019

30. Bolli GB. Physiological insulin replacement in type 1 diabetes mellitus. *Exp Clin Endocrinol Diabetes* 2001;109(Suppl. 2):S317–S332

31. Gong WC. Determining effective insulin analog therapy based on the individualized needs of patients with type 2 diabetes mellitus. *Pharmacotherapy* 2008;28:1299–1308

32. Lantus [package insert]. Bridgewater, NJ, Sanofi-Aventis U.S. LLC, 2019

33. Rosenstock J, Davies M, Home PD, et al. A randomized, 52-week, treat-to-target trial comparing insulin detemir with insulin glargine when administered as add-on to glucose-lowering drugs in insulin-naïve people with type 2 diabetes. *Diabetologia* 2008;51:408–416

34. Dornhorst A, Luddeke H-J, Sreenan S, et al. Safety and efficacy of insulin detemir in clinical practice: 14-week follow up data from type 1 and type 2 diabetes patients in the PREDICTIVE™ European cohort. *Int J Clin Pract* 2007;61:523–528

35. Levemir [package insert]. Princeton, NJ, Novo Nordisk Inc., 2019

36. Toujeo U-300 [package insert]. Bridgewater, NJ, Sanofi-Aventis U.S. LLC, 2020

37. Blair HA, Keating GM. Insulin glargine 300 U/mL: a review in diabetes mellitus. *Drugs* 2016;76:363–374

38. Lau IT, Lee KF, So WY, et al. Insulin glargine 300 U/mL for basal insulin therapy in type 1 and type 2 diabetes mellitus. *Diabetes Metab Syndr Obes* 2017;10:273–284

39. Bergenstal RM, Bailey TS, Rodbard D, et al. Comparison of insulin glargine 300 U/mL and 100 U/mL in adults with type 1 diabetes: continuous glucose monitoring profiles and variability using morning or evening injections. *Diabetes Care* 2017;40:554–560

40. White JR. Advances in insulin therapy: a review of new insulin glargine 300 U/mL in the management of diabetes. *Clin Diabetes* 2016;34(2):86–91

41. Heller S, Buse J, Fisher M, et al. Insulin degludec, an ultra-longacting basal insulin, versus insulin glargine in basal-bolus treatment with mealtime insulin aspart in type 1 diabetes (BEGIN Basal-Bolus Type 1): a phase 3, randomised, open-label, treat-to-target non-inferiority trial. *Lancet* 2012;379: 1489–1497

42. Tresiba [package insert]. Plainsboro, NJ, Novo Nordisk Inc., 2019

43. Schloot NC, Hood RC, Corrigan SM, et al. Concentrated insulins in current clinical practice. *Diabetes Res Clin Pract* 2019;148:93–101

44. Kalra S. High concentration insulin. *Indian J Endocrinol Metab* 2018;22: 160–163

45. De la Peña A, Seger M, Soon D, et al. Bioequivalence and comparative pharmacodynamics of insulin lispro 200 U/mL relative to insulin lispro (Humalog®) 100 U/mL. *Clin Pharm Drug Dev* 2016;5(1):69–75

46. Humulin R U-500 [package insert]. Indianapolis, IN, Lilly USA, LLC, 2019

47. Grunberger G, Bhargava A, Ly T, et al. Human regular U-500 insulin via continuous subcutaneous insulin infusion versus multiple daily injections in adults with type 2 diabetes: the VIVID study. *Diabetes Obes Metab* 2020;22(3):434–441

48. Lenhard J, Rockwell K, Tran K. A uniform approach in the use of U-500 regular insulin in the management of patients with obesity and insulin resistance: the clinician's view. *Del Med J* 2017;89(5):142–146

49. Bergen PM, Kruger DF, Taylor AD, et al. Translating U-500R randomized clinical trial evidence to the practice setting: a diabetes educator/expert prescriber team approach. *Diabetes Educ* 2017;43(3):311–323

50. Humalog Mix 75/25 [package insert]. Indianapolis, IN, Lilly USA, LLC, 2012

51. Humalog Mix 70/30 [package insert]. Indianapolis, IN, Lilly USA, LLC, 2019

52. Novolog Mix 70/30 [package insert]. Princeton, NJ, Novo Nordisk Inc., 2007

53. Humulin 70/30 [package insert]. Indianapolis, IN, Lilly USA, LLC, 2019

54. Novolin 70/30 [package insert]. Plainsboro, NJ, Novo Nordisk Inc., 2019

55. Ryzodeg 70/30 [package insert]. Plainsboro, NJ, Novo Nordisk Inc., 2019

56. Rotenstein LS, Ran N, Shivers JP, Yarchoan M, Close KL. Opportunities and challenges for biosimilars: what's on the horizon in the global insulin market. *Clin Diabetes* 2012;30(4):138–150

57. Heinemann L, Hompesch M. Biosimilar insulins. *J Diabetes Sci Technol* 2014;8(1):6–13

58. U.S. Food and Drug Administration. FDA statement: statement on efforts to help make development of biosimilar and interchangeable insulin products more efficient [article online]. Available from https://www.fda.gov/news-events/press-announcements/statement-efforts-help-make-development-biosimilar-and-interchangeable-insulin-products-more. Accessed 26 April 2020

59. Yamada T, Kamata R, Ishinokachi K, et al. Biosimilar vs originator insulins: systematic review and meta-analysis. *Diabetes Obes Metab* 2018;20(7): 1787–1792

60. Admelog [package insert]. Bridgewater, NJ, Sanofi-Aventis U.S. LLC, 2019

61. Basaglar [package insert]. Indianapolis, IN, Lilly USA, LLC, 2019

62. Frid A, Hirsch L, Gaspar R, et al. New injection recommendations for patients with diabetes. *Diabetes Metab* 2010;36:S3–S18

63. Del Prato S. In search of normoglycaemia in diabetes: controlling postprandial glucose. *Int J Obes Relat Metab Disord* 2002;26(Suppl. 3):S9–S17

64. Hanefeld M, Temelkova-Kurktschiev T. Control of post-prandial hyperglycemia—an essential part of good diabetes treatment and prevention of cardiovascular complications. *Nutr Metab Cardiovasc Dis* 2002;12:98–107

65. Hofman PE, Derrak JBG, Pinto TE, et al. Defining the ideal injection techniques when using 5-mm needles in children and adults. *Diabetes Care* 2010;32:1940–1944

66. Diabetes Control and Complications Trial (DCCT) Research Group. Implementation of treatment protocols in the Diabetes Control and Complications Trial. *Diabetes Care* 1995;18:361–375

67. American Diabetes Association. 9. Pharmacologic approaches to glycemic treatment: *Standards of Medical Care in Diabetes—2021. Diabetes Care* 2021;44(Suppl. 1):S111–S124

68. Danne T, Deiss D, Hopfenmuller W, et al. Experience with insulin analogues in children. *Horm Res* 2002;57(Suppl. 1):46–53

69. Davidson J. Strategies for improving glycemic control: effective use of glucose monitoring. *Am J Med* 2005;118(Suppl. 9A):27s–32s

70. Ruben RR, Peyrot M, Kruger DF, et al. Barriers to insulin injection therapy. *Diabetes Educ* 2009;35:1014–1022

71. Peyrot M, Rubin RR, Kruger DF, et al. Correlates of insulin injection omission. *Diabetes Care* 2010;33:240–245

Diabetes Technology: Continuous Subcutaneous Insulin Infusion, Continuous Glucose Monitoring, and Automated Insulin Delivery Systems

---

Highlights
Diabetes Technology: Continuous Subcutaneous Insulin Infusion, Continuous Glucose Monitoring, and Automated Insulin Delivery Systems

■ Insulin therapy by continuous subcutaneous insulin infusion (CSII), also referred to as insulin pump therapy, approximates physiological insulin delivery by continuously delivering a basal rate of rapid-acting insulin together with bolus insulin administration before meals.

■ For the motivated and capable patient with the necessary resources, insulin pump therapy is indicated for
  • suboptimal glycemic control,
  • wide blood glucose excursions,
  • dawn phenomenon with elevated fasting blood glucose levels,
  • nocturnal hypoglycemia,
  • frequent severe hypoglycemia,
  • pregnancy or pre-pregnancy planning,
  • gastroparesis,
  • day-to-day variations in schedule that are not well managed by multiple insulin injections, or
  • patient preference for more flexibility.

■ The basal rate should consist of 40–50% of the patient's total daily insulin dose. With traditional insulin pumps, several different basal rates can be set in a 24-h period to accommodate diurnal variations in insulin sensitivity.

■ Meal boluses are usually calculated based on carbohydrate content, using an individual insulin-to-carbohydrate ratio of 1 unit of insulin per a specific number of grams of carbohydrate, usually 1 unit of insulin for every 7–15 g carbohydrate for adults and, for example, 1 unit of insulin for every 20–30 g carbohydrate for children or insulin-sensitive adults.

■ The patient's insulin sensitivity factor or correction factor, which describes the effect of 1 unit of insulin on a patient's blood glucose level, is used to compute the correction dose of insulin that will bring premeal or between-meal hyperglycemia to glycemic target range, which is typically set at 100–120 mg/dL. The insulin sensitivity factor is individualized and is calculated using a variety of formulas (e.g., 1,500/total daily dose).

■ Patients can be taught to make additional adjustments in the basal rate or bolus size for illness, exercise, and menses.

■ Risks of continuous subcutaneous insulin infusion include

- skin infections, which can be avoided or resolved with regular changes of the infusion set every 2–3 days, by keeping the infusion site clean and dry, and by removing the infusion set at the first signs of discomfort or redness;

- unexplained hyperglycemia, usually resulting from a partial or complete interruption of insulin delivery that, if untreated, can lead to diabetic keto-acidosis; and

- hypoglycemia, which can be reduced by monitoring blood glucose levels at least four times per day and weekly at 2:00–4:00 A.M, in individuals who are not augmenting pump therapy with continuous glucose monitoring and always before operating a motor vehicle or using hazardous machinery.

■ The insulin pump should be worn at all times. The patient should use an alternative insulin regimen if the pump is removed for >1–2 h.

■ Successful insulin pump therapy requires thorough and ongoing education in technical components of the insulin pump and skills needed to adjust insulin for variations in daily activities.

■ Insulin pump therapy in combination with a continuous glucose monitor (sensor augmented insulin pump) can improve blood glucose control without increasing hypoglycemia.

■ Hybrid closed-loop automated insulin delivery systems are now available and are continuously being refined with the goal of improving the time spent in target range (70–180 mg/dL), without an increase in hypoglycemia, while aiming to minimize the self-care burden involved in intensive diabetes management.

■ The future of diabetes treatment is promising thanks to advanced technologies that could lead to better information management systems, further improvements in insulin pumps, and closed-loop insulin delivery systems.

Diabetes Technology: Continuous Subcutaneous Insulin Infusion, Continuous Glucose Monitoring, and Automated Insulin Delivery Systems

The search for optimal insulin regimens led to the development of technology, such as continuous subcutaneous insulin infusion (CSII) via use of an insulin pump, which helps patients achieve diabetes self-management goals. Insulin infusion pumps deliver insulin continuously in a manner that approximates physiological insulin delivery and provides flexibility in day-to-day diabetes management. Along with continuous glucose monitoring (CGM), insulin pumps assist patients with diabetes to achieve near-normal glycemic control.

CONTINUOUS SUBCUTANEOUS INSULIN INFUSION

CSII includes a small pump, about the size of a beeper or cell phone, that contains a reservoir of rapid-acting (insulin lispro, insulin aspart, insulin glulisine) or faster-acting insulin aspart. Most patients today use rapid-acting insulin in their insulin pumps. After filling the reservoir with a 2- to 3-day supply of the prescribed insulin, the reservoir is connected to an ~18- to 43-inch length of plastic tubing. At the end of the tubing is a 25- to 29-gauge needle or a soft Teflon cannula that the patient inserts into the subcutaneous tissue at a 30- to 45-degree or a 90-degree angle, depending on the type of infusion set used.

The exception to this is the Omnipod pump, which is tubing free and is referred to as a "patch pump." It has a built-in infusion cannula in the insulin reservoir or pod for insertion into the subcutaneous tissue. With the Omnipod pump, the patient injects insulin into the pod before placement on the skin and insertion of the infusion needle. The pod has a self-adhesive backing that attaches to the skin. The pod, like the infusion sets used with other pumps, must be changed every 2–3 days; a built-in alarm warns patients when the 72-h mark is approaching. Patients use a remotely connected personal diabetes management (PDM) system, which is now available as a smartphone-like device (Omnipod DASH) to remotely control the on-body pod to deliver insulin boluses.

All insulin pumps deliver insulin in two ways. Basal insulin delivery is optimized to control hepatic glucose production and maintain stable glucose concentrations when the patient is fasting. In practice, most patients achieve glycemic goals using multiple different basal rates over a 24-h period. Depending on the model, insulin pumps can deliver basal rates from 0.025 to 35 units/h (in 0.025- to 5.0-unit increments).

Insulin is also delivered as a bolus in anticipation of a meal or to correct hyperglycemia. Depending on the pump manufacturer, the pump can deliver a 0.025- to

80-unit bolus (most deliver a maximum of 25–35 units) in 0.025- to 2-unit steps. Insulin pumps can be programmed to deliver a bolus over a longer period of time, referred to as an extended or square-wave bolus. For example, a patient may program their pump to deliver 4 units over a 3-h period to accommodate snacking (such as at a party) or for a high-fat meal. Patients also can program a combination of both a standard bolus and square-wave or extended bolus at the same time, also referred to as a dual-wave or combination bolus, typically used for high-fat and/or high-protein meals.

Insulin infusion pumps have therapeutic and safety features that facilitate achieving treatment goals in different situations. Depending on the pump manufacturer, patients can use their pumps to achieve several goals, including the following:

■ Program different insulin-to-carbohydrate ratios (ICRs), different insulin sensitivity factors (ISFs), and different blood glucose targets by time of day.

■ Use the pump's bolus calculator to determine insulin bolus requirements at mealtime and also to correct hyperglycemia. Most pumps calculate the amount of correction-dose insulin depending on the time and amount of the previous insulin bolus to prevent stacking or overlapping doses of insulin. This specific feature is referred to as "active insulin time" or "insulin on board." Use of these in-built bolus calculators should be encouraged as they eliminate the need for the patient to manually make these complex and time-consuming calculations and reduce risk of stacking insulin boluses.

■ Program several basal rate patterns (two to seven, depending on the pump model) so the patient can easily switch, for example, from a weekday to weekend pattern, perimenstrual to postmenstrual pattern, high- to low-activity pattern, or day- to night-shift pattern.

■ Temporarily adjust the basal rate for periods of increased physical activity, illness, or stress without changing the usual basal rate program. The user can set the temporary basal rate in units or as a percentage of the usual basal rate.

■ Suspend basal delivery if necessary. It is advised not to suspend for longer than 1 h at a time, to reduce the risk of rebound hyperglycemia.

■ Review the amounts and times of previous boluses, which can be a valuable feature to avoid "stacking" of boluses and related hypoglycemia.

■ Program boluses via a variety of shortcut options that bypasses having the user access the normal bolus screen.

■ Set a missed meal bolus alert to remind patients to bolus for a meal. This is an important feature for patients who frequently forget to administer insulin boluses before meals.

■ Set reminders on the pump to check blood glucose levels at specific times of day or recheck blood glucose if is was previously above or below a specified level.

Some insulin pumps are watertight or water-resistant so that patients can wear their pumps while showering or engaging in some water sports, and this can be a practical consideration for some patients when choosing a particular pump. The size of the insulin reservoir varies in different pump types, and the total daily insulin requirements of the patient can be an important factor when choosing pumps.

BENEFITS OF CONTINUOUS SUBCUTANEOUS INSULIN INFUSION

CSII leads to less dose-to-dose variability in insulin absorption than injections, and because of this, CSII is associated with less glycemic variability and modestly reduces the risk of hypoglycemia.[1,2] In practice, appropriately programmed basal infusion rates may allow patients to skip or delay meals and maintain more stable glycemic control during periods of changing insulin sensitivity. The ability to discreetly administer multiple meal insulin boluses without the need for multiple injections can be a valuable convenience for more prolonged meals in restaurants or on social occasions. The ability to deliver meal boluses over an extended time can be a valuable feature for patients with gastroparesis or when consuming high-fat and/or high-protein meals that are associated with delayed gastric emptying and increased insulin requirements in the late postprandial period.

Basal infusion rates are usually programmed to coincide with anticipated diurnal variation of insulin sensitivity. Patients often need lower basal rates during the night (between ~11:00 P.M. and 3:00 A.M.) and higher basal rates between 3:00 or 4:00 A.M. and 9:00 A.M. to offset the effect of the dawn phenomenon and to prevent an increase in blood glucose levels in the morning. The basal rate can be adjusted temporarily during exercise, during the post-exercise period when hypoglycemia is likely to occur, during illness, or before and during menses when insulin requirements tend to be higher.[3]

Insulin pump therapy optimizes the conditions for achieving good glycemic control while maintaining lifestyle flexibility.[4] This therapeutic approach provides patients with the opportunity to fully participate in their self-care because they can make decisions about and adjustments to aspects of the regimen on a moment-to-moment basis as they encounter varying aspects of daily life.

Proper patient selection is critical to ensure the success of insulin pump therapy (see Table 7.1). Consider patients for insulin pump therapy

- to improve or stabilize glycemic control, especially if multiple daily insulin regimens have failed to solve self-management problems, such as wide glycemic excursions, nocturnal or frequent hypoglycemia, and effects of the dawn phenomenon;
- to increase lifestyle flexibility and deal with day-to-day variations in work or exercise schedule; or
- to meet increased self-management needs (i.e., to allow greater participation in self-care).

Patients who have erratic schedules, work different shifts, or travel frequently also can benefit from insulin pump therapy.

Table 7.1 — Patient Selection Criteria for Continuous Subcutaneous Insulin Infusion

- Medical and metabolic indications, including
  - Suboptimal glycemic control using multiple daily injections
  - Wide blood glucose excursions
  - Different day versus night basal insulin requirements, including the dawn phenomenon
  - Frequent severe hypoglycemia
  - Nocturnal hypoglycemia
  - Pregnancy or planned conception
  - Gastroparesis
  - Variable daily schedule or lifestyle not well managed with multiple daily injections
- Patient demonstrates the technical and physical ability to
  - Perform blood glucose monitoring accurately and frequently
  - Perform the technical components of insulin pump use
  - Absence of serious disease or disability (e.g., visual impairment, poor dexterity) that would impair technical performance
- Patient demonstrates the intellectual ability to
  - Learn both the technical and cognitive components of pump use (e.g., meal planning, the meaning of blood glucose levels, how to adjust insulin doses)
  - Determine the relationship between aspects of the regimen (e.g., food and insulin, activity, blood glucose levels)
- Patient demonstrates the motivation to
  - Perform frequent glucose monitoring to detect "unexplained" hyperglycemia, in particular to troubleshoot in the event of unexplained hyperglycemia that could be indicative of an insulin pump failure
- Patient needs ongoing follow-up appointments for therapy optimization
- Patient has the financial resources or a source of reimbursement for insulin pump, blood glucose monitoring supplies, and ongoing healthcare

INITIAL DOSAGE CALCULATIONS FOR INSULIN PUMP THERAPY

Rapid-acting insulin has a quicker onset of action and a shorter duration of action than regular insulin. Rapid-acting insulin should be administered 15 min before ingestion of a meal, although to achieve optimal postprandial control, some higher glycemic index foods are best covered if the bolus is taken even earlier. The more rapid onset and peak activity of the rapid-acting insulin can hasten correction of hyperglycemia and lessens the likelihood that boluses taken close together will have overlapping action, leading to hypoglycemia (insulin "stacking"). Recently, faster-acting insulin aspart (Fiasp) was approved by the U.S. Food and Drug Administration (FDA) in October 2019 for use in insulin pumps, and recommendations for dosing through a pump are similar to other rapid-acting insulin analogs (see Chapter 6, Multicomponent Insulin Regimens).

BASAL INSULIN DOSAGE

Most patients with type 1 diabetes (T1D) require basal rates in the range of 0.4–2.0 units/h, with the average basal rate being 0.7–0.9 unit/h. The average total daily dose (TDD) for adults is 0.5–1.0 unit/kg body wt/day. Children typically require similar TDD unless they have substantial residual insulin secretion, which may occur soon after diagnosis or in the "honeymoon." Adolescents typically require a TDD of at least 1.0 unit/kg.

To calculate starting basal rate, reduce pre-pump TDD by 10–25%. If the patient has a history of problematic hypoglycemia or hypoglycemia unawareness, it usually is prudent to be even more aggressive with dosage reductions.

For example, a patient with a hemoglobin A_{1c} (A1C) level of 7.2% takes a TDD of insulin of 55 units (reduce by 20%: 55 units × 0.20 = 11 units). Reduce the TDD to 44 units (55 − 11) and divide by 2 (total basal dose should be 50% of TDD: 44 units ÷ 2 = 22 units). Divide the total basal dose by 24 h (22 units ÷ 24 h = 0.92 unit/h). The starting basal dose for this patient is 0.9 unit/h.

An alternative method to calculate the total daily basal dose is to multiply the patient's weight in kilograms by 0.3–0.5. If the patient's weight is 176 lb (80 kg), the basal rate would be calculated as follows: (80 kg × 0.3 unit/kg) ÷ 24 h = 1.0 unit/h.

Before initiating pump therapy, ideally try to eliminate intermediate-acting insulin 12–24 h, long-acting insulin 24 h, and ultra-long-acting 36–48 h prior to starting basal insulin delivery. Instruct patients to take injections of short- or rapid-acting insulin, as needed, every 3–4 h to keep blood glucose levels reasonably controlled until pump therapy is begun.

Patients using insulin pump therapy have the advantage of programming different basal rates for varying diurnal insulin needs. When initiating pump therapy, it is often simplest to begin with a single basal rate for the entire 24-h period (e.g., 0.9 unit/h all day). However, patients often need lower basal rates between bedtime and 3:00 A.M. and higher basal rates between 3:00 and 9:00 A.M. to deal with the dawn phenomenon. Patients may need an intermediate basal rate during the rest of the day. Adjustment of the basal rate should be done in increments of 10–20% at a time. Using the previous example, if the patient's blood glucose profile or CGM tracings revealed these varying diurnal insulin needs, the basal rate profile at initiation might be

- from 11:00 P.M. to 3:00 A.M., 0.9 unit/h;
- from 3:00 A.M. to 7:00 A.M., 1.2 units/h; and
- from 7:00 A.M. to 11:00 P.M., 1.0 unit/h.

Evaluate the basal rate by closely evaluating 24-h CGM tracings, or for patients who are using self-monitoring of blood glucose (SMBG) alone, by evaluating the 3:00 A.M. and fasting blood glucose levels and asking the patient to perform basal check tests (i.e., omission of a meal with glucose checks performed every 2 h for a specific duration of time, usually 4–6 h). If these values are higher or lower than desired, adjust the basal rate accordingly, usually by increments of 0.05–0.2 unit/h. If the 3:00 A.M. and fasting blood glucose levels are widely discrepant, the patient may need different basal rates during sleep and in the early morning (before waking) hours. Adjust the daytime basal rate based on basal check tests. For example, if the patient develops hypoglycemia when meals are skipped or delayed, the daytime basal rate is too high. In practice, changes in basal insulin infusion rates can take up to 60–90 min or longer to affect blood glucose concentrations, and this delay needs to be factored into the timing for adjustments of basal infusion rates (e.g., recurrent hypoglycemia occuring at 3:00 A.M. suggests the need to decrease the basal rate starting at 2:00 A.M. or sooner).

In those patients who are already using CGM systems, glucose patterns may further help guide the distribution of basal insulin delivery over the 24-h period without the need for overnight glucose checks or basal check tests; for example, high glucose values beginning to rise in the early morning are suggestive of dawn phenomenon, whereas a consistent pattern of glucose drifting downward in middle of the afternoon suggests setting a lower basal rate during this period.

BOLUS INSULIN DOSAGE

As a starting point, in optimizing prandial insulin dosing, bolus doses are calculated based on the number of grams of carbohydrate consumed. Preferably, the patient starting a pump has demonstrated competence in counting carbohydrates before the initiation of pump therapy. Ultimately, the goal is for the patient to be able to match the meal boluses to the intake of carbohydrate at each meal and snack with an individualized ICR.

During the first few days or weeks of pump therapy, it is useful to ask the patient to follow a prescribed meal plan based on the patient's usual dietary intake to establish the patient's ICR. It may be preferable to do this before initiating insulin pump therapy while the patient is still using a multiple daily insulin injection regimen. Ask patients to keep detailed food records to help them master carbohydrate counting skills, demonstrate their ability and motivation to estimate carbohydrate intake, and determine their insulin-to-carbohydrate needs. Begin with a prescribed insulin dose for the meal plan and make adjustments until blood glucose levels are in the desired range. In some individuals, dietary fat and protein can have a substantial effect on mealtime insulin requirements. Therefore, in practice, meals used to determine the patient's ICR ideally should be low fat and low protein.

In the absence of CGM augmentation, frequent blood glucose monitoring must be performed to determine the effectiveness of insulin dosages relative to accurate carbohydrate counting and bolus calculations and to the patient's usual activity level. Blood glucose monitoring should be done, initially, before each meal, within 1–2 h after the start of each meal, at bedtime, and at 2:00–4:00 A.M. until glycemic goals are achieved. Further adjustments will be required as the patient implements the insulin regimen under various situations.[5]

The patient's ISF is used to adjust boluses to correct for premeal and between-meal hyperglycemia. To estimate the patient's ISF, divide 1,500 or 1,800 by the TDD. For example, a patient whose TDD is 46 units has an ISF of 40 mg/dL based on the following equation: $1{,}800 \div 46$ units = 39 mg/dL (round up to 40 mg/dL).

One unit of rapid-acting insulin is expected to decrease this patient's blood glucose by 40 mg/dL. Begin with a conservative estimate of the ISF to minimize hypoglycemia. In general, patients who have diurnal changes in basal insulin requirements and different ICR for breakfast, lunch, and dinner will also require a different ISF for different time periods in the day. In practice, if basal insulin requirements during the dawn period are increased, the need for correction insulin dosages also will increase (i.e., lower ISF) during this time period.

Conversely, if the basal insulin requirements during the early nocturnal period are lower, a corresponding need for correction insulin dosages also will decrease (i.e., higher ISF) during this time period.

When determining the amount of supplemental insulin, if the pump is programmed to calculate the bolus needs based on the patient's ISF, it will compute the insulin dose needed based on the time of the most recent bolus (i.e., active insulin or insulin on board) to prevent stacking or overlapping insulin doses. For adults the typical starting insulin duration time is programmed at 4 h. If hypoglycemia from dose stacking is a problem, then the duration of action in the pump should be even longer. This is of particular relevance in patients with chronic kidney disease or high titer insulin antibodies, where the insulin pharmacokinetics/dynamics may be prolonged. If a patient chooses to give a manual bolus or overrides the bolus calculator, and if using regular insulin and the last bolus was taken <4 h ago, some percentage of activity from that bolus remains; therefore, reducing the supplemental insulin dose with that in mind is appropriate (about 25% per hour). With rapid-acting insulin, peak pharmacodynamic activity is achieved in ~100 min, but the duration is still a concern if the patient is calculating a between-meal correction bolus.

Calculations of meal dosing and correction dosing are automated by the bolus calculator as long as glucose and carbohydrate content data is entered by the patient. Combining the ICR with the ISF, a patient with an ICR of 1 unit/10 g carbohydrate and an ISF of 1 unit/40 mg/dL would calculate a premeal bolus as follows (assuming the previous bolus was given beyond the programmed duration of insulin):

Blood glucose target is 110 mg/dL
ISF = 40
Blood glucose level = 179: 179 – 110 (target blood glucose) = 69;
    69 ÷ 40 (correction dose = 1.725 units)
Carbohydrate intake = 60 g: 60 ÷ 10
    (ICR is 1 unit/10 g) = 6 units of insulin
Calculated total bolus is 6 + 1.7 = 7.7 units

INSULIN DOSAGE ADJUSTMENTS

DIET

Patients need to learn to adjust insulin boluses for variations in dietary intake so that blood glucose levels remain in the desired range. Typically, 1 unit of insulin will cover 10–15 g carbohydrate. This can range from 0.5 to 2.0 units for every 10–15 g carbohydrate in patients with T1D. Patients, with the help of their clinician, will use food and glucose monitoring records to optimize the ICR, which may vary depending on the time of the meal (more insulin is often required at breakfast and less at lunch) or the type of food eaten (more insulin for same amount of carbohydrate is often required if combined with protein and fat). Precise estimates of the patient's insulin needs can be determined using detailed food, insulin, and blood glucose records, reviewed over a few days to a few weeks, when initiating intensive therapy. Periodic review and reassessment of a patient's ICR and pump settings in general should be performed, especially in the setting of growth, changes in weight, intercurrent illness, new medications and changes in physical activity.

A unique beneficial feature of insulin pump therapy is that it provides the user the option to alter the bolus duration in a variety of different ways. A square-wave or extended bolus can be used when eating small amounts of food over an extended period of time, such as at a banquet or cocktail party, or when eating meals containing more slowly digested (lower glycemic index) carbohydrates such as beans or legumes. The use of a square-wave or extended bolus may ensure better postprandial coverage in patients with gastroparesis. Patients can also program a normal bolus and square-wave or extended bolus at the same time (dual-wave or combination bolus). This approach might be useful for coverage of higher fat foods, such as pizza, that are characterized by delayed gastric emptying and late postprandial insulin resistance from free fatty acids.[6] Research indicates that these meals are optimally covered by a combination bolus consisting of 10–50% initially with the remainder delivered over 2–3 h.[7] To compensate for the insulin resistance from the free fatty acids, the total insulin dose will need to be more than that given for a meal with similar carbohydrate but lower total fat content. There are considerable interindividual differences in the amount of additional insulin that should be given for higher fat meals; in practice, it is prudent to start with ~30% dose increase which may be delivered over 2 h with 50% delivered immediately and the other 50% extended over the 2-h period. Further dose adjustments for future higher fat meals may be required based on a retrospective review of postprandial glucose profiles.[8]

EXERCISE

CSII allows for greater flexibility in insulin dosing adjustments around exercise than multiple-dose injection (MDI) therapy.[3] The use of a temporary basal dose reduction feature allows patients to minimize the need for carbohydrate intake around exercise, thereby allowing patients to more effectively use exercise as a strategy for weight control. Dosing adjustments need to be individualized based on the type, duration, and strenuousness of the activity.[9] In general, decrease the premeal bolus by 25–50% for moderate levels of planned aerobic activity within 3 h of a meal. When exercising for sustained periods (>60 min), the patient may need to program a temporary basal rate reduction of 20–70% starting 60–90 min before exercising. At the conclusion of the exercise when muscle glucose uptake decreases, the blood glucose may increase because of ongoing accelerated hepatic glucose production resulting from the reduced basal insulin levels. The immediate reinstitution of basal insulin following exercise can be important in preventing this rebound hyperglycemia. Use of a temporary reduction in the basal rate after exercise also can be an effective strategy to avoid post-exercise hypoglycemia that often occurs several hours after exercise.

Many pumps offer the ability to use a different set of 24-h basal rates that are most effective for exercise. For example, for planned exercise at specific times, the patient may choose to switch to his or her exercise-day program, which the patient presets with lower basal rates at specific times.

ILLNESS

Because hyperglycemia and ketosis from interruption of insulin delivery is often accompanied by nausea and abdominal discomfort, train patients who are beginning pump therapy that whenever they have a deterioration in metabolic control associated with physical symptoms, they must troubleshoot for insulin nondelivery (see the next section). For patients who take oral steroids, the basal rates of the pump can be adjusted to match the pharmacologic action of the steroids, thereby facilitating better glucose control than can be achieved using MDI. For example, if the patient is taking prednisone in the morning, basal rates from midmorning through late afternoon or early evening, as well as the meal and correction bolus doses for lunch and dinner programmed into the pump bolus calculator, would be increased.

RISKS OF CONTINUOUS SUBCUTANEOUS INSULIN INFUSION

SKIN INFECTION

Skin infections can occur at the infusion site and range from a small area of mild inflammation and tenderness to a frank abscess.[10] Antibiotics usually completely resolve the infections. Large abscesses may need to be surgically incised and drained.

To avoid infection, patients should keep the infusion site clean and dry at all times. Alcohol swabs or soap and water usually are adequate to cleanse the skin before needle insertion. Patients who experience recurrent infusion site infections may need to use antibacterial cleansers. Known carriers of *Staphylococcus aureus* require antibacterial cleansers and meticulous care of the infusion site. Patients should be instructed to remove moist tape and to clean and dry the area around the needle insertion site. This procedure is especially important during the summer heat or during increased physical activity.

Insertion of cannulas in areas with visible lipohypertrophy, scar tissue, stretch marks, or areas where the underlying tissue feels hard should be avoided because these areas are usually associated with poor or unpredictable insulin absorption. Use of alternative nonscarred sites should be encouraged.

There are several types of infusion sets with various cannula and needle types, including straight or angled needles, needles attached to an adhesive disk, Teflon cannulas with needle introducers, and steel needles. Pump infusion sets can be placed in the abdomen, hip, thigh, upper buttock, or upper arm. In practice, the abdomen is often the most comfortable site. Because exercise can enhance insulin absorption, patients who are physically active may benefit from avoiding placement of the infusion catheter on an exercising limb. Teflon cannulas come in 6- to 17-mm lengths. Patients have a choice of cannula length and angle insertion, depending on their body type. Angled Teflon sets are less prone to kinking than perpendicular Teflon sets, especially in patients who are thin and have limited subcutaneous fat. In practice, the use of insertion devices with angled sets (such as the Sil-serter) sometimes will lead to erratic insulin absorption, and angled sets are best inserted by hand. In contrast, use of insertion devices with perpendicular sets is not associated with this problem, and inserters are a valuable convenience that can enable patients to place infusion sets in areas such as the upper buttock that cannot be readily reached manually. Most cannula or infusion site problems, such as difficulty with needle insertion and skin breakdown, can be resolved by finding the type of cannula and tape or adhesive that best suits the individual patient. For patients who have frequent hyperglycemia resulting from the interruption of insulin delivery because of kinking of the Teflon infusion catheters, use of a metal needle catheter can provide a practical solution.

Most infusion sets have self-adhesive tape; use of an additional adhesive dressing or surgical tape can help secure the needle or cannula and tubing in place. If patients are allergic to the self-adhesive infusion sets, find a tape or surgical dressing that does not cause a skin reaction, or have the patient apply a protective solution or dressing (I.V. Prep Antiseptic Wipes, Tegaderm, Skin-Tac, Bard Protective Barrier Film, Mastisol, or Skin Bond) before inserting the infusion set.

UNEXPLAINED HYPERGLYCEMIA AND KETOACIDOSIS

Because the insulin pump only uses rapid- or short-acting insulin, even a partial interruption of insulin delivery can rapidly result in hyperglycemia. Complete interruption of insulin delivery can result in ketosis or ketoacidosis within a few hours.

Patients new to insulin pump therapy must be taught to consider the possibility of interrupted insulin delivery any time high blood glucose levels persist for no apparent reason. There are many potential causes of unexplained hyperglycemia or ketoacidosis related to partial or complete failure of some component of the insulin infusion pump, tubing, or infusion set or pod (see Table 7.2). When a patient encounters a high blood glucose level (>250 mg/dL) that cannot be explained by an alteration in a component of the treatment plan (e.g., illness, food indiscretion, missed insulin bolus), the patient should administer a correction bolus, and if the blood glucose level has not decreased within 2–4 h should complete a systematic investigation of the pump, cartridge or reservoir, infusion set or pod, infusion site, and insulin to identify the cause and rule out interruption of insulin delivery. If urine ketones are also present or blood ketone (β-hydroxybutyrate) levels are increased, disruption of insulin delivery must be considered. A correction bolus should be administered using an insulin syringe, and not via the pump, and then the patient should troubleshoot the infusion system. If the patient detects a problem with the site, the infusion set tubing, or the connection between the reservoir and the infusion set, immediately change the cannula or pod and site. If a problem with the pump is identified, reprogram the pump or contact the pump manufacturer to troubleshoot the problem or replace the pump if it is within the warranty period.

Table 7.2—Unexplained Hyperglycemia: Factors to Consider

- ■ Insulin pump
  - • Basal rate programmed incorrectly
  - • Battery depleted
  - • Pump malfunction
  - • Cartridge or reservoir does not advance properly or pod is not functioning
  - • Program or pump alarms
  - • Program functions cannot be set
- ■ Cartridge or reservoir
  - • Improper placement in the pump
  - • Empty cartridge or reservoir (insulin depleted)
  - • Leakage of insulin
  - • Cartridge or reservoir not positioned to advance and infuse
  - • Did not prime reservoir or infusion set correctly
- ■ Infusion set and needle or cannula
  - • Insulin leakage
  - • Dislodged needle, cannula, or pod
  - • Bent or kinked cannula or incorrect cannula or pod insertion
  - • Insulin not administered to account for dead space after introducer needle is removed when infusion cannula is inserted
  - • Air in infusion set tubing
  - • Blood in infusion set tubing
  - • Occlusion at the site
  - • Infusion set in place >48–72 h
  - • Tear in the tubing
  - • Occlusion of the insulin in the infusion set
  - • Loose cartridge or reservoir and infusion set connection
- ■ Infusion site
  - • Redness, irritation, inflammation, induration
  - • Discomfort
  - • Placement in an area of hypertrophy or scar tissue
  - • Placement in an area of friction or near the belt line
- ■ Insulin
  - • Has clumped particles or crystallized appearance
  - • Is beyond expiration date
  - • Was exposed to extreme temperatures
  - • Vial has been used for >1 month or is nearly empty
  - • Prior bolus inadequate for carbohydrate consumed

If the patient administers an insulin bolus via a conventional syringe and the blood glucose level improves, the problem is with the insulin pump or the reservoir or pod, and not with the insulin.

Loss of potency of insulin should be suspected if no improvement in blood glucose levels are seen when the patient administers insulin via syringe and/or changes the reservoir and infusion set.

If no obvious cause is found, assume that there is an infusion problem, most likely caused by kinking of the infusion set or scarring of the infusion site. Replacing the pump reservoir and infusion set or pod and changing the site is recommended. If the pump is inoperable or malfunctioning, patients should resort back to a multiple daily injection regimen until the pump can be replaced (see Chapter 6). All patients should know how to use an alternative insulin regimen with insulin syringes in case a problem with the pump or some component of the infusion system occurs. Instruct patients to always carry extra insulin pump supplies (batteries, infusion sets, and pump cartridges, syringes, or pods), and insulin syringes or an insulin pen delivery device. In case of hospitalization, it is best to be prepared to carry in these supplies, in case the hospital policy will permit self-management to continue, under the conditions of the hospitalization and as long as the patient is capable and willing to continue safe device operation while hospitalized.[11]

When the patient detects unexplained hyperglycemia and corrects the problem, the patient should also treat hyperglycemia and ketonuria. The patient should monitor blood glucose and urine or blood ketone levels every 1–3 h. Advise the patient to take insulin boluses in amounts determined by the patient's insulin sensitivity and daily insulin requirements until urine ketones have cleared (or blood ketone levels are <0.6 mmol/L) and blood glucose levels have returned to the desired range. The patient who develops nausea and vomiting and is unable to maintain fluid intake should go to an emergency department for evaluation and treatment.

HYPOGLYCEMIA

A lower incidence of hypoglycemia has been observed with insulin pump therapy as compared with multiple daily injections.[4] Strategies to avoid hypoglycemia and methods of teaching hypoglycemia awareness are essentially the same for any intensive diabetes management approach, regardless of the mode of insulin delivery. Patients should have a source of rapidly absorbed carbohydrate, such as juice, regular soda, or glucose tablets, with them at all times, including at work, in the car, at the gym, and at the bedside. Encourage patients to check their blood glucose levels before operating machinery or a motor vehicle. All patients using a pump should have glucagon and a close family member or friend instructed on its use. To avoid accidentally infusing insulin, advise patients to disconnect the infusion set tubing before removing a used cartridge or reservoir or replacing an infusion set. The patient should not use the prime, load, or fill tubing feature while an infusion set is connected to the body. Another major issue that can contribute to risk for hypoglycemia in pump users is incorrectly set basal rates, in particular, inadvertent increases in basal rates to cover food-related elevations in the blood glucose. For example, patients noticing consistent elevations in their blood glucose levels in the late evening period because of snacking commonly will increase the basal rates rather than take additional bolus insulin; however, on occasions when evening eating is delayed or food intake is less, hypoglycemia will occur.

Avoiding severe hypoglycemia begins with selecting patients who are good candidates for intensive therapy (see Tables 7.1 and 7.3) and by consideration of sensor-augmented and closed-loop insulin delivery systems (see below). Patients must be prepared to check blood glucose levels four or more times a day and/or use their continuous glucose monitor for the vast majority of the time to monitor device operation and to make and evaluate decisions regarding insulin doses.

Table 7.3—Education for Insulin Pump Therapy

Phase 1: Choosing insulin pump therapy (one or two outpatient visits)

- Components of insulin pump therapy
- Advantages and disadvantages of insulin pump therapy
- Financial requirements
- Goals of therapy
- Carbohydrate counting
- Suitability for insulin pump use (this can include a several-month trial of frequent blood glucose monitoring, trial of multiple daily insulin injections, carbohydrate counting, and use of insulin sensitivity or correction factor)

Phase 2: Initiating insulin pump therapy

- Several sessions with healthcare team over several months, a technical training session with pump trainer, and a visit with healthcare provider
- Technical components of the insulin pump (see Table 7.4)
- Blood glucose–monitoring technique and accuracy confirmed
- Carbohydrate counting review and fine-tuning skills to establish ICR
- Symptoms, prevention, and treatment of hypoglycemia
- Optional trial of wearing the insulin pump using normal saline
- Determination of initial starting basal rate

Phase 3: Post initiation of insulin pump therapy

- Frequent phone contact for 7–10 days and biweekly follow-up visits for first 2–4 weeks; maintain close contact for 2–6 months; have patient keep food, blood glucose, and insulin records
- Focus on mastering blood glucose monitoring, calculating meal boluses based on carbohydrate counting, calculating correction bolus doses based on glucose monitoring, and insulin pump operation
- Fine-tune insulin dosages to achieve blood glucose goals
- Identify relationships between blood glucose readings and food intake, activity, and insulin
- Adjust aspects of the regimen to meet lifestyle needs based on patient input
- Assist patient to integrate the treatment plan into daily life

Ongoing follow-up

- Continuing visits every 1–3 months of 30–60 min duration using all team members as needed
- Interpreting blood glucose readings
- Adjusting insulin for variations in dietary intake and activity
- Using the pump and advanced pump options to deal with varying situations
- Dealing with pump-related problems
- Adapting treatment recommendations to changes in lifestyle
- Anticipating situations that could cause alterations in glycemic control
- Identifying obstacles to implementing treatment recommendations and developing strategies to overcome obstacles
- Setting and evaluating treatment and blood glucose goals

Patients often take insulin without checking their blood glucose levels, a practice that increases the risk of hypoglycemia. This should be discouraged. Patients should be encouraged to carry their blood glucose testing equipment with them at all times. Physical capabilities to program the pump and monitor its operation are necessary; patients must be able to understand the relationships between components of the treatment plan and their effects on blood glucose levels. Anticipating insulin needs for varying activities increases the likelihood that patients will make the appropriate adjustments in insulin so that blood glucose levels remain in the desired range.

WEARING THE PUMP

During patient training, it needs to be reinforced that the pump must be worn at all times. Removing the pump for >1–2 h without insulin supplementation puts the patient at risk for developing hyperglycemia and ketosis. Patients frequently are concerned about initiating insulin pump therapy because they believe that it will interfere with activities they enjoy. The pump can be worn during most activities, with the exception of contact sports. Because of the effect of heat on insulin stability, pumps should not be submerged in hot tubs and should not be exposed to high temperatures during long periods of time outdoors during the summer. If the pump is not watertight, it must be removed for showering or placed in a plastic sheath. If engaging in certain water sports, the patient can remove the pump or place the pump in a waterproof holder. Some pumps are watertight for unlimited surface activity and are considered watertight only up to certain water depths and for specified periods of time.

Most patients are concerned about what to do with the insulin pump during sexual activity, but they may not feel comfortable asking about it. If the patient does not bring up the topic, initiate a discussion about sexual activity and pump use. Most couples find that wearing the insulin pump during sexual activity does not interfere with sexual intimacy. If the pump is disconnected during sexual activity, caution the patient to resume insulin pump delivery within an hour or so. After sexual activity, check the tape and infusion set or pod to ensure that the system is intact and secure. Following are alternatives for patients who do not wish to wear their pumps for certain periods of time, including days at the beach, vacations, or an evening out:

- If using an infusion set with a disconnect feature, disconnect the pump for up to 1–2 h depending on the level of activity (leave the needle or cannula in place).
- Take injections of rapid- or short-acting insulin before meals and wear the pump at night to provide basal insulin needs; or take an injection of basal insulin to cover most basal insulin requirements during the day when the pump is removed, and use the pump for boluses and to provide additional basal coverage for the dawn period.

Remind patients that there are some limitations on the timing of insulin and meals while off the pump. More blood glucose monitoring should be performed while using an alternative insulin regimen.

When traveling by air, patients usually do not have problems with airport security while wearing an insulin pump. Patients may request a letter from their healthcare provider that documents their need for an insulin pump, pump supplies, and blood glucose monitoring equipment. Because patients cannot carry liquids, such as juice or soda, through airport security, they should carry glucose tablets and then purchase juice or soda after getting through security, if necessary. Patients who have very tightly controlled blood glucose levels should be aware that changes in altitude have been shown to cause unintended insulin delivery from their pumps.[12] During takeoff, when cabin air pressure decreases, pumps can deliver additional insulin, whereas during descent the converse can occur.

PATIENT EDUCATION FOR CONTINUOUS SUBCUTANEOUS INSULIN INFUSION

Appropriate education for insulin pump therapy takes place in three phases (see Table 7.3). The first phase occurs before initiating pump therapy. During this period, discuss the advantages and disadvantages of pump therapy, the patient's personal treatment goals, and the patient's resources to successfully manage insulin pump therapy. As indicated, initiate strategies to establish the patient's suitability for insulin pump use, such as a trial of performing and recording four blood glucose tests per day, using a multiple daily insulin regimen with carbohydrate counting, or adding insulin algorithms to an existing insulin regimen before establishing the patient's ISF. With the healthcare provider's assistance, the patient should choose the pump brand and model and verify insurance coverage and requirements. For example, before approving an insulin pump, some insurance companies require several weeks or months of blood glucose records and an A1C level.

After the decision to initiate insulin pump therapy is made, the second phase of education begins. During this period, verify blood glucose–monitoring and nutrition knowledge and self-management skills. This education can be accomplished through a series of outpatient visits with certified diabetes educators. The patient can be given the opportunity to wear a pump for several days, using normal saline to master the technical skills associated with pump therapy and to increase his or her comfort with wearing a pump. Most pump initiations are done on an outpatient basis and the patient will need to perform frequent blood glucose monitoring and maintain close contact with the healthcare team. This contact usually consists of frequent phone calls or faxing or e-mailing blood glucose or CGM results, carbohydrate counting, and bolus dose records. Focus on teaching the basic components of insulin pump therapy, including the technical components of the pump (see Table 7.4), the pump's insulin delivery system, carbohydrate counting, monitoring blood glucose, and preventing and treating hypoglycemia and hyperglycemia.

Table 7.4 — Technical Components of Insulin Pump Therapy

- ■ Pump operation
  - • Placement of the battery or batteries
  - • Programming the meal bolus and extended or square-wave bolus
  - • Programming basal rates
  - • Preparation and placement of insulin cartridge or reservoir and infusion set or pod (priming infusion set)
  - • Infusion site selection, rotation, and care
  - • Meaning of alarms and how to respond
  - • Programming additional basal rates and basal rate programs as needed and temporary basal rate changes
  - • Programming additional pump options (e.g., beep or vibrate, bolus calculator, quick bolus options, setting alarms, history features)
  - • Troubleshooting
- ■ Self-monitoring of blood glucose
  - • Determining proper technique
  - • Confirming accuracy of results
  - • Interpreting blood glucose readings
  - • Setting blood glucose goals
  - • Using linked meter to help calculate required insulin dosages based on personal settings
- ■ Carbohydrate counting and learning relationship between insulin and food
- ■ Using insulin sensitivity or correction factor
- ■ Learning about hypoglycemia and hyperglycemia: symptoms, causes, prevention, and treatment
- ■ Learning about unexplained hyperglycemia: causes, prevention, identification, and treatment
- ■ Managing sick days
- ■ Dealing with exercise
- ■ Determining options for special occasions
- ■ Deciding on an insulin regimen when insulin pump use is not desired or pump malfunctions
- ■ Determining decision-making strategies for dealing with lifestyle changes

The third phase begins after insulin doses are determined and the patient demonstrates technical competence using the pump. This phase is an intensive period of follow-up lasting 2–6 months, during which time the patient masters the skills learned in the second phase and integrates those skills into the usual activities of daily life. Visits with a member of the healthcare team may take place every 2–3 weeks in addition to frequent phone contact. The patient should keep blood glucose and food records to facilitate learning to quantify food and plan meals and to identify relationships among blood glucose levels, insulin dose and timing, dietary intake, and activity. These records also enable the healthcare team to modify insulin doses and determine whether the patient understands all of the components of the treatment plan. Some issues to consider when educating the patient with erratic glucose control are listed in Table 7.5.

Table 7.5—Practical Issues to Consider in the Pump Patient with Erratic Glucose Control

Several pump-specific issues can cause erratic glucose control in the pump user. In the course of follow-up visits, the clinician should routinely:

1. Examine pump infusion sites. Scarring and lipohypertrophy of infusion sites are not uncommon causes for unpredictable glucose levels, especially in long-term pump users.
2. Ask whether the patient has had catheter kinking or dislodgement. Plastic catheters that are inserted perpendicular to the skin surface are more prone to kink or become dislodged, especially with activity and perspiration. Solutions include use of antiperspirants or changing to metal needle infusion sets, plastic sets with a shorter cannula, or other types of plastic infusion sets that are less prone to kinking. These include sets that insert obliquely such as the Silouette and VariSoft. Note of caution: Practical experience indicates that use of insertion devices with oblique catheters often is associated with erratic glucose control, presumably because of tissue trauma; patients should be encouraged to insert these oblique catheters manually. Patients using Teflon catheters who have inexplicable glucose fluctuations should be offered a trial with a metal needle catheter.
3. Ask whether the patient changes the pump reservoir and infusion system on a regular basis. This can be confirmed with the pump download. In reviewing the pump and glucose data, check for the tendency for elevated and erratic glucose in the period preceding infusion set changes. Insulin instability in the pump infusion system can manifest as higher glucose levels if the reservoir and catheter is kept in place for too long or even as precipitation in the infusion system. Practical experience indicates that some patients with erratic glucose levels who are prescribed a change in insulin type or more frequent catheter and infusion system changes will demonstrate improved glycemic control.[13] Routines need to be individualized, however, and some patients with stable and good glycemic control can safely use reservoirs and catheters for longer than mandated by the label.

Review of pump downloads can help identify the possible causes for erratic glucose levels. In reviewing the data, the clinician should

- check priming history of the pump to assess how frequently the infusion system is being changed, and examine whether delayed set changes are associated with increased glucose levels;
- check percentage of basal to bolus insulin—a high percentage of basal insulin in the patient with frequent hyperglycemia may suggest that bolus doses are being missed, whereas a high percentage of basal insulin in the patient with frequent hypoglycemia may indicate that basal rates are too high and are contributing to the hypoglycemia; and
- check bolus history to detect possible missed meal boluses and also determine whether boluses are being delivered to correct hyperglycemia.

CONTINUOUS GLUCOSE MONITORING

CGM devices measure glucose concentration in the subcutaneous interstitial fluid every 1–5 min via a short subcutaneous enzyme-tipped electrode or fluorescence technology (glucose sensor).

The most common CGM devices include a transcutaneous sensor attached to an on-body transmitter, which is linked wirelessly to a handheld receiving device (receiver or reader), which displays the glucose data for the patient to review. A subcutaneous implantable CGM with on-body transmitter, currently approved for use for 90 days in the United States and 180 days in Europe, is also available (Eversense, Senseonics). The implantable sensor requires a minor surgical procedure to insert and remove the sensor by a trained healthcare professional, unlike for all other available CGM systems, which allow self-insertion by the user.

Receivers can be either standalone devices or integrated into insulin pumps, mobile phones, or certain smart watches. Interstitial glucose readings are displayed either in real time (RT-CGM) or on demand when a patient chooses to intermittently scan or wave the reader over the sensor (intermittently scanned/flash CGM [IS-CGM]).

RT-CGM devices automatically display glucose readings at regular, 5-min intervals and utilize real-time data to generate alarms and alerts, which include the glucose value generating the alert, which is subsequently automatically transmitted to the linked receiving device.

Alerts are generated when sensor glucose levels reach predefined thresholds, set by users along with their clinician, and can help detect and predict hypoglycemia and hyperglycemia and can alert the patient to rapidly changing glucose levels.

IS-CGM (FreeStyle Libre 1 and 2, Abbott Diabetes Care) automatically measures glucose levels every minute and stores readings every 15 min; however, it displays interstitial glucose levels only when a patient scans the sensor. Each time the patient scans the sensor, the reader graphically displays the trajectory of predicted future glucose levels and the previous 8 h of retrospective glucose values. The original Libre system, which is still available, does not include audible or vibratory alarms that alert a patient to glucose excursions in real time. In 2020, the FDA approved the Libre 2 system, which includes optional real-time high and low glucose alerts. However, unlike RT-CGM, the patient still needs to scan the sensor to review the actual blood glucose value that triggered the alert.

BENEFITS OF USING CONTINUOUS GLUCOSE MONITORING

RT-CGM has become a routine part of intensive management in adults and children with T1D and is now regarded as being an integral part of the standard of care in this population.[14]

Several trials have demonstrated the positive impact of the use of RT-CGM on reduction in A1C along with reduction in hypoglycemia.[15-18] RT-CGM has been shown to be of similar benefit to people with T1D on multiple daily injections and insulin pump users.[17] Moreover, people with T1D with very tight glycemic control often rely on CGM to maintain excellent control and mitigate hypoglycemia. In addition, significant improvements in subjective well-being and treatment satisfaction has also been reported.[19]

Early CGM systems were prescribed as adjuncts to self-monitoring of blood glucose and insulin dosing based off of CGM data was not approved. However, given the increasing accuracy of CGM systems, in 2016, the FDA began approving CGM use for insulin dosing decisions, independent of SMBG, starting with the Dexcom G5 CGM system.

The insights gained from CGM about postprandial glucose patterns can help optimize diabetes management. For example, higher glycemic index carbohydrate breakfast foods (such as cold cereal) lead to a rapid postprandial glucose spike, and uncovering this pattern will focus attention on the need for early premeal bolusing or even prompt a change to alternative lower glycemic index breakfast foods. Some patients will overreact to postprandial glucose spikes identified by the CGM by taking excessive additional insulin boluses, and the resultant insulin dose stacking can lead to hypoglycemia. During the initial training when patients start on RT-CGM, they should be cautioned about the risks from overbolusing and about the need to consider residual insulin on board from the premeal bolus before taking additional insulin.

There is currently less robust data to support the use of CGM in people with type 2 diabetes (T2D).[1] However, the evidence base is growing and studies have reported reduction of A1C in people on oral antihyperglycemic medications, basal insulin alone, and multiple daily dose insulin therapy.[20]

In addition, recent reports have confirmed glycemic and nonglycemic benefits in pregnant women with T1D on CSII as well as MDI therapy.[21] During pregnancy, maintenance of tight maternal blood glucose concentrations at or near normoglycemic levels is required to reduce adverse maternal, fetal, and neonatal outcomes.[22] Some of the reported nonglycemic and neonatal benefits of CGM in pregnancy include a reduction in large-for-gestational-age infants, shorter hospital and neonatal intensive care unit length of stay, and lowered rates of neonatal hypoglycemia. The role of CGM in women with gestational diabetes and pregnant women with T2D is supported by very limited data.[23]

There are currently no guidelines for the use of CGM in the inpatient setting. Use of certain medications such as acetaminophen and frequent inpatient clinical scenarios, including hypoxemia, hypotension or hypothermia, and fluid overload, may interfere with accuracy. However, recent data suggest that in-hospital use of RT-CGM in patients with insulin-treated T2D may mitigate the risk of hypoglycemia.[24] Moreover, during the COVID-19 pandemic, in-hospital CGM has been widely employed, with early publications suggesting noninferiority to SMBG.[25] However, further studies are needed to assess the accuracy and role of CGM in the hospital setting.[26]

DIFFERENCES BETWEEN CONTINUOUS GLUCOSE MONITORING SYSTEMS: REAL-TIME, INTERMITTENTLY SCANNED, AND PROFESSIONAL

RT-CGM devices automatically display glucose readings at regular 5-min intervals and utilize real-time data to generate alarms and alerts. To use RT-CGM technology safely and effectively, patients need to develop advanced diabetes self-management skills and must understand several key concepts (including physiologic lag). Currently available CGM devices measure glucose in the interstitial fluid in the subcutaneous tissue, whereas glucose meters measure capillary blood glucose obtained by fingerstick. When the glucose concentration is changing, there is a physiologic lag in the equilibration of glucose between these two compartments. This lag has important implications for the interpretation of data from CGM and the use of RT-CGM in diabetes self-management. Currently, RT-CGM does not completely eliminate the need for fingerstick capillary blood glucose measurements (SMBG), although as improvements in CGM accuracy and reduction in physiological lag time improve, the exact role of SMBG in CGM users continues to evolve.[27]

The alarms for hypo- and hyperglycemia are an important feature of RT-CGM devices. To ensure that the patient derives maximum benefit from use of the alarms, the alarm thresholds must be individualized. If alarm thresholds are set at the "ideal" level (e.g., low = 90 mg/dL, high = 180 mg/dL), the patient will be warned of most low and high glucose values; however, they also will experience frequent false alarms with increased risk for "alarm burnout" and a related tendency to ignore the alarms. Conversely, if alarm thresholds are set more widely (e.g., low = 60 mg/dL, high = 240 mg/dL), the patient will experience few false alarms and less risk for alarm burnout, but they will not be warned about all low and high glucose values. During clinic follow-up visits, review alarms thresholds to determine whether the patient is getting the necessary alarms when the glucose is low, especially during the nocturnal period when vulnerability to hypoglycemia is the greatest. Ideally, alarms for low glucose should go off prior to developing symptoms of hypoglycemia, to help prevent over treatment and consequent rebound hyperglycemia. If the patient is having frequent, intermittent fasting hyperglycemia but the high alarm is not going off, the high alarm threshold may need to be reduced.

In order to obtain a full 24-h glucose profile, users of IS-CGM (Freestyle Libre, Abbott Diabetes Care) must scan at least every 8 h to avoid gaps in the glycemic data collection. This could be problematic for patients who tend to sleep longer than 8 h and in patients who are forgetful or distracted by competing life demands.[28]

IS-CGM and many modern RT-CGM systems are factory calibrated; therefore, SMBG is not required for calibration and glucose data integrity. However, in certain circumstances sensor glucose values may not be accurate, and SMBG to confirm a sensor glucose value or to calculate insulin doses is recommended. Examples of these circumstances include a sensor value that is not consistent with symptoms of hypoglycemia or hyperglycemia, or to confirm restoration of euglycemia shortly after treatment of a hypoglycemic event.

The differences between IS-CGM and RT-CGM should be discussed with patients to help select systems that are most suited to an individual patient's circumstances. Certain patients prefer to receive the real-time alerts, and alerts may be preferable for patients who experience impaired hypoglycemic awareness. However, some patients may find the amount of data generated by RT-CGM overwhelming and may find the alerts and alarms to be a nuisance and potentially anxiety provoking.

Professional CGM is a term used for clinic-owned CGM systems that allow intermittent, retrospective, diagnostic glucose data review. Professional CGM differs from personal CGM in three ways: *1*) CGM data are typically not available for patients to view in real time (masked or blinded), although certain systems do allow the clinician to "unmask" the real-time data flow to allow the patient to view the CGM tracings in real time if they choose. In blinded mode, the patient is possibly less likely to alter an aspect of their lifestyle or make unusual treatment decisions based on the data. *2*) It is typically only worn for 3–14 days, depending on the clinical scenario and device. *3*) There are **no** alarms to warn of hyperglycemia or hypoglycemia when patients are using it in blinded mode. Data resulting from intermittent short periods of CGM wear can provide helpful information on glycemic patterns, including nocturnal hypoglycemic episodes that may be missed with routine SMBG data review. Retrospective review of CGM data, especially if contextualized with patient diaries, including exercise and meals, can provide further insightful information to support therapy adjustments and review the impact of lifestyle modifications and choices on glucose patterns.

WEARING A CONTINUOUS GLUCOSE MONITOR

CGM systems are fairly easy to use as insertion systems have become more user-friendly over time. Allergic reactions to skin adhesives have been reported. The risk of developing subcutaneous scar tissue and skin infections while wearing a CGM is lower than reported with insulin pump insertion sets. It is important to recognize and emphasize to patients, that in order to derive maximum benefit, they should wear their CGM devices for as much time as possible.[15] Patients who wear their own personal devices consistently for at least 6 out of every 7 days derive the most benefit. Patients should be encouraged to keep CGM receivers or smartphones within earshot, respond to all alerts, and frequently look at their CGM tracings. The wealth of CGM data is only as good as the individual patient's response to these data. Incorporating CGM data into treatment decisions and self-management skill takes times and all CGM users should be thoroughly educated and supported by the diabetes care team. In particular, it is important to assess a patient's dexterity and visual acuity to ensure they are capable of inserting a transcutaneous sensor and reading CGM data on receivers.

CONTINUOUS GLUCOSE MONITORING TERMINOLOGY AND CLINICAL TARGETS

As discussed in Chapter 5, recent consensus has been attained pertaining to the standardization of CGM metrics and definitions of glycemic targets.[29] Common CGM-derived metrics include time in range (TIR), time below range (TBR; or hypoglycemia), time above range (TAR; or hyperglycemia), glucose management indicator (GMI), and coefficient of variation (CV).

For most individuals with T1D and T2D, the recommended target TIR is the time spent between sensor glucose values of 70 and 180 mg/dL (TIR^{70-180}). Different TIR targets exist for different patient populations (see Chapter 5 and Table 5.1).

Hypoglycemia, or TBR, is classified in three levels:

- Level 1: sensor glucose between ≥54 mg/dL and 70 mg/dL
- Level 2: sensor glucose <54 mg/dL independent of presence of symptoms of hypoglycemia
- Level 3: episode of severe hypoglycemia, defined as a hypoglycemic event characterized by altered mental and/or physical status requiring assistance from a third party independent of the glucose value

Hyperglycemia, or TAR, is similarly classified in three levels:

- Level 1: sensor glucose >180 mg/dL and <250 mg/dL
- Level 2: sensor glucose >250 mg/dL
- Level 3: sensor glucose >250 mg/dL with positive ketones

For every additional 10% (2.4 h/day) spent in TIR^{70-180}, A1C reductions of approximately 0.8% may be expected.[30] Although there is a wide range of associated A1C values associated with various percentiles of time spent in range, a good rule is that 50% TIR^{70-180} corresponds with an A1C of approximately 8%, and 70% TIR^{70-180} corresponds to an A1C of approximately 7%.

Targets must be individualized, and current consensus recommendations for patients with diabetes and greater risk of hypoglycemia favor a more conservative approach to reduce the risk of hypoglycemia. In particular, in the older and/or high-risk population, defined as people with cognitive deficits, cardiovascular disease, osteoporosis, increased risk of falls, renal disease, and individuals requiring assistance with diabetes care, less stringent goals should be considered as follows:

- TBR <70 mg/dL should not exceed <1% (or ~15 min/day)
- TIR^{70-180} and TAR are more relaxed with goals of TIR >50% and TAR >50% (>180 mg/dL) with up to 10% time spent >250 mg/dL being acceptable

Average glucose measured by CGM may be used to calculate the GMI, which is an estimate of A1C, as long as at least 70% of the data is available (minimum of 10 days of wear out of 14 days). While often closely approximating a laboratory A1C, it may differ from laboratory A1C. The recent GMI nomenclature has been developed to highlight the difference between CGM-derived glucose averages and laboratory A1C.[31] Discrepancies between A1C and GMI highlight the well-known limitations of the A1C, particularly in individuals living with chronic kidney disease, anemia, and hemoglobinopathies.

Glycemic variability is an important and often overlooked aspect of intensive diabetes management.[32] It represents the glycemic excursions. When glycemic variability is elevated, there is an increased risk of both hypo- and hyperglycemia. A high degree of variability also may be associated with vascular diabetes complications and impaired quality of life. CGM provides patients and clinicians with the best opportunity to assess and address heightened glycemic variability. There are multiple definitions and methods to assess glycemic variability, but it may be defined as the CV (standard deviation/average glucose) and is expressed as a percentage. The lower the CV, the lower the glycemic variability. A CV <36% has been agreed upon as a reasonable goal for patients with T1D, but lower CV goals may be reasonable for patients with T2D.

CONTINUOUS GLUCOSE MONITOR INTERPRETATION

Before starting to review CGM data, it is important to ensure adequate data collection. It has been shown that 14 days of data collection and derived metrics is strongly correlated with laboratory A1C. As a result, it is often not necessary to review more than 14 days of data at a time unless unusual circumstances in the last 14 days (illness, use of glucocorticoids) are likely to skew the data.

Data are displayed as aggregates over the time frame set for analysis into a single, 24-h "modal" day, in which all collected data over multiple days are collapsed and plotted according to time (without regard to date) as if they occurred over 24 h. This presentation (the ambulatory glucose profile [AGP]) enables clinicians to quickly identify the time(s) of day when glucose is most consistently low or high and when the most variability is occurring. Curves representing the median (50th), 25th and 75th (interquartile range [IQR]), and 5th and 95th frequency percentiles are also presented to help quickly identify glucose variability over the 24 h. The IQR provides an easy visualization of glucose variability, whereas the CV is a useful measure to assess glucose stability and changes in variability over time. The closer the interquartile curves are to the median, the less glucose variability is present and the less likely the patient is at risk of hypoglycemia, whereas the farther apart the interquartile curves are from the median, the higher the glucose variability and the greater the risk of hypoglycemia. In some patients, glucose variability may differ during different times of the day. Recognition of this may help guide diabetes self-management. The daily glucose profiles present thumbnail or calendar view profiles of the 24-h pattern for each day that is included in the overall profile. This allows for comparison of patterns on specific days (e.g., weekend versus weekday) and permits a more comprehensive discussion with patients regarding special circumstances that may be responsible for extremes or fluctuations in glucose readings.

The one-page AGP is an excellent place to begin data review and patient discussion because it allows for a visual representation of most of the important CGM metrics in a single document.[33] All currently available CGM systems incorporate the AGP into their reporting software. When reviewed with the patient, the AGP creates an opportunity for education and increased patient involvement in diabetes self-management.

After reviewing the AGP, clinicians should focus next on time spent in hypoglycemia, assess whether any episodes of severe hypoglycemia occurred, and clarify whether an episode of hypoglycemia occurred while not wearing the CGM system. Any episodes of hypoglycemia occuring while wearing the CGM should prompt exploration of alarm and alert audibility, the context of the episode, and potential contributing factors. A plan to mitigate future episodes should be developed during the visit. If hypoglycemia occurs while not wearing the CGM, possible causes of gaps in therapy should be discussed. Among the potential causes of gaps in therapy include challenges with insurance coverage, diabetes burnout, and alarm fatigue. Assessing whether any patterns can be observed at specific times of day or specific days of the week allows the clinical team to address potential causes such as exercise (including commuting by walking, scheduled gym/exercise classes, cleaning the house, shift work).

Periods of hyperglycemia should be reviewed next. Hyperglycemia occuring at consistent times of day or specific days of the week should prompt identification of potential causes such as uncovered food intake, ICR and/or sensitivity factor maladjustment, or fear of hypoglycemia, particularly if hyperglycemia is consistent throughout the day and/or overnight.

Glycemic variability (standard deviation and/or CV) is another important CGM-derived metric that should prompt discussion of possible causes given that elevated glycemic variability is associated with hypoglycemic risk. Clinicians should assess in a nonjudgmental way how often an insulin dose may have been forgotten. Inconsistent adherence to insulin therapy may contribute to glycemic variability.

The GMI may create some confusion when it differs significantly from the laboratory-measured A1C. For example, consider the patient whose GMI is lower than his or her A1C; sensor glucose average is 124 mg/dL, GMI is 6.6%, and laboratory A1C is 7.2%. In this case the clinician should confirm that the time spent in hypoglycemic range is not excessive. A personalized plan to mitigate hypoglycemia may need to be implemented and increasing the patient's A1C goal may need to be considered.

Alternatively, another patient may have a sensor glucose average and GMI greater than A1C; for example, sensor glucose average is 160 mg/dL and GMI is 7.4%, whereas A1C is 6.8%. In this case the focus should be directed to the time spent in hyperglycemic range, and intensification of therapy may be required to improve glucose control and a lower A1C target should be set. Moreover, someone who has an A1C of 8.0% and who spends 10% of the day in hypoglycemic range would benefit from a diabetes management plan that differs from someone who has an A1C of 8.0% and only spends 1% of the day in hypoglycemic range.

ALERTS, ALARMS, AND RATE OF CHANGE

CGM provides a dynamic glucose tracing that includes the current glucose level along with trend arrows predicting the rate and directionality of glucose change. It also provides threshold alerts for low and high blood glucose values and for the rise and fall rate of sensor glucose. Most CGM systems have the capability to set alerts for specific glucose levels and for defined rate of change in glucose levels to help to mitigate hypoglycemia and hyperglycemia. Moreover, an alarm for a predefined urgent low is built in to many CGM systems and cannot be turned off, thereby potentially mitigating severe hypoglycemia.

It is essential to inform patients early on when starting to use CGM data for diabetes self-care of the differences between SMBG and CGM glucose data: from the static fingerstick value—a "point in time"—to the dynamic sensor glucose value along with its with trend arrow, the latter helping to "anticipate" future glucose levels.[34]

The alerts for hypo- and hyperglycemia are an important feature of RT-CGM devices. To ensure that the patient derives maximal benefit from use of the alarms, the alarm thresholds must be individualized. In a person with T1D with glucose values ranging from low to 200 mg/dL, alert thresholds should be considered to be set at low = 80 mg/dL and high = 180 mg/dL. The patient will be warned of most low and high glucose values and he or she will act upon them as needed. In a patient with glucose values ranging from 120 mg/dL to 300 mg/dL, low alert may be set at 100 mg/dL and high at 280 mg/dL to avoid alerts occurring too often. In fact, if alerts are set too tightly, the pateint will be warned often with frequent alerts that over time may result in potential alarm burnout and the related tendency to ignore the alarms, as well as the potential for over-bolusing insulin to respond to high glucose alerts and subsequent hypoglycemia. Conversely, if alarm thresholds are set too widely (e.g., low = 60 mg/dL, high = 240 mg/dL), the patient will experience few false alarms and less risk for alarm burnout; however, he or she will not be warned about all low and high glucose values with potential reduction in the benefit of use of CGM. Of note, some patients may benefit from the use of CGM independent of the use of alerts that may exacerbate or trigger anxiety around glucose management. A low alert set at 80 mg/dL is a good starting point for most patients given that it is not quite in the hypoglycemia range but will often warn ahead of an episode and help prevent the onset of undesirable symptoms of hypoglycemia.

During initial training, when patients first start on RT-CGM, they should be advised to passively observe and learn from all the new data gathered by the CGM for the first few days/weeks and avoid acting upon them. In particular, they should be cautioned about the risks of overreacting by administering too many insulin boluses to correct previously unrecognized postprandial hyperglycemia as well as to avoid overcorrection of hypoglycemia due to the lag time it may take for the CGM to display the rise in sensor glucose level (~20 min). Patients should also be warned and prepared that many more glucose values will be available as compared to SMBG (12 glucose readings per hour for SMBG versus 288 glucose readings per day for CGM).

CGM data provide significant insight into postprandial glucose patterns that can help optimize diabetes management. For example, higher glycemic index carbohydrate breakfast foods (such as cold cereal) lead to a rapid postprandial glucose spike, and uncovering this pattern will help patients and clinicians focus attention on the need for early premeal bolusing or suggest a change to alternative lower glycemic index breakfast foods (i.e., whole wheat bread/high fiber cereals). High-fat meals (e.g., pizza) lead to a slow and prolonged rise in glucose followed by a prolonged postprandial hyperglycemic period lasting several hours. Uncovering this pattern may help to focus on the need for an increase in the amount of insulin required, which may be administered split into 2 doses a few hours apart by injection or delivered as a combination bolus via pump.

Trend arrows add further information on glucose patterns. The directionality of trend arrows allows individuals to anticipate glucose levels projected about 30 min into the future. This additional information can then be used proactively to adjust insulin dose or preemptively treat impending hypoglycemia. Upward trend arrows indicate rising glucose levels and may suggest a need for additional insulin; downward trend arrows indicate falling glucose levels and may suggest a need for less insulin, if bolus of insulin is planned, or corrective action with carbohydrate intake to avoid hypoglycemia. Adjustment in insulin dose based on trend arrows should be performed when planning to have a meal.

Steady state is a flat arrow suggesting that glucose levels are not increasing/decreasing more than 1 mg/dL each minute. However, symbols used for trend arrows differ among different CGM systems. Whereas rising and falling arrows (oblique/up or downtrend) are suggestive of a more rapid change in glucose level, different manufacturers use oblique, up- or downward one or two arrows to refer to different rates of change ranging from 1 to 3 mg/min (Fig. 7.1).

There is a physiologic lag in the equilibration between glucose values in the bloodstream and the interstitial fluid compartments. A lag of several minutes can be observed leading to discrepancies between SMBG and CGM values. For example, if a patient just ate a meal and blood glucose is rising, SMBG may read higher than CGM because absorption of nutrients will raise glucose faster in the bloodstream than interstitial fluid. On the other hand, after exercise, glucose uptake into muscle from interstitial fluid will happen first, reduction in blood glucose levels will occur slightly later, and CGM glucose will read lower than SMBG. This lag time has important clinical implications, in particular during treatment of hypoglycemia or hyperglycemia. Patients should be instructed, if in doubt, to confirm resolution of hypoglycemia by performing SMBG.

Considering the directionality of trend arrow before bolusing for meals may be encouraged for more experienced CGM users to allow for modification in the

↑ ↑	Blood glucose is rising >3 mg/dL per minute
↑	Blood glucose is rising 2–3 mg/dL per minute
↗	Blood glucose is rising 1–2 mg/dL per minute
→	Blood glucose is changing <1 mg/dL per minute
↘	Blood glucose is falling 1–2 mg/dL per minute
↓	Blood glucose is falling 2–3 mg/dL per minute
↓ ↓	Blood glucose is falling >3 mg/dL per minute

Figure 7.1—Dexcom G5 receiver trend arrows.

insulin dose depending on the trajectory of glucose rise or fall. For example, if a particular patient is planning to eat 40 grams of carbohydrate and uses an ICR of 1:10 and sensitivity factor of 1:50 with target glucose set to 110 mg/dL, and the sensor glucose value is 110 mg/dL and trending up by 2 mg/dL/min, the estimated glucose level in 30 min will be ~60 mg/dL greater than at the time of bolus. The patient may consider adding 1 extra unit to the 4 units administered to cover the meal to mitigate hyperglycemia. Conversely, if the trend arrow is trending down by 2 mg/dL/min the estimated glucose in 30 min will be ~60 mg/dL lower. The patient may consider reducing the insulin bolus by 1 unit to mitigate hypoglycemia.

Many recent CGM devices on the market are factory calibrated; therefore, there is no need to perform SMBG to ensure optimal functioning. However, some CGM systems require at least 2 calibrations per day, 12 h apart. The best time to calibrate is during glucose steady state, denoted by a flat arrow.

In March 2018, Dexcom G6 was the first CGM designated as an integrated continuous glucose monitoring (iCGM) system for determining blood glucose levels in children aged 2 years and older and adults with diabetes. The Freestyle Libre 2 CGM followed as the second iCGM device, approved in individuals aged 4 years and older. This type of CGM system is permitted by the FDA to be used as part of an integrated system with other compatible medical devices and electronic interfaces, which may include automated insulin dosing systems, insulin pumps, blood glucose meters, or other electronic devices used for diabetes management.

CGM data can be projected to other devices such as smartphones, smart wristwatches, and computers with the possibility of sharing data safely with clinicians, spouses, and others remotely. Some CGM devices (Dexcom G5, Dexcom G6, and Eversense) offer the ability to share real-time glucose data with family members, caregivers, and clinicians. This capability is particularly valuable for parents and caregivers of pediatric patients, patients living in group homes, partners of people traveling for work, and elderly people and their caregivers. The share features allows significant others/caregivers to remotely monitor and receive alerts and alarms throughout the 24 h. Moreover, clinicians can access data remotely, using cloud-based tracking of the most recent CGM recorded data, allowing for quick data review over the phone or via televisit without having to download or be physically present in clinic. Of note, data gathered in this scenario are not real time but have a 3-h time lag.

AUTOMATED INSULIN DELIVERY SYSTEMS

Increasing integration of insulin pumps and CGM has become available over the last few years. Early systems simply allowed CGM data to be viewed directly on pump screens. Subsequent iterations have allowed CGM glucose inputs to begin to automatically modulate basal insulin delivery controlled by an algorithm in the pump. These systems automatically and continually modulate basal insulin delivery based on a variety of different in-built computer algorithms reacting to real-time sensor glucose levels. More recent versions have allowed for sensor-augmented pumps to automatically suspend basal insulin delivery upon a threshold sensor glucose value and to resume insulin delivery once glucose levels begin to normalize. Later iterations allowed automated suspension of basal insulin based on a predicted future low glucose event. In this iteration, automated basal insulin reduction and/or suspension began prior to hypoglycemia onset, further reducing the risk of clinically significant hypoglycemia. The most recent versions in clinical use today allow for algorithm-controlled automatic basal insulin delivery so that basal insulin increases as well as decreases based on sensor glucose inputs. However, patients are still required to manually administer prandial and correction boluses (hybrid closed-loop [HCL] approach).

Two HCL systems are currently available on the U.S market: Medtronic Minimed 670G and Tandem t:slim X2 with Control-IQ.[35] The Minimed 670G HCL system was FDA approved in 2016 as the first HCL system and uses the Medtronic Guardian CGM.[36] The system automatically adjusts basal insulin every 5 min based on an algorithm that analyzes the patient's insulin requirement over the last 48 h to 1 week. The pump basal rate is driven by a proportional–integral–derivative algorithm with insulin-on-board feedback. It does not use traditional preset basal doses entered into the pump when running in hybrid closed loop (auto mode). However, preset basal doses are necessary to revert to when the pump is not being driven by the algorithm and is running in open loop (manual mode). Patients are required to manually administer mealtime and correction boluses if sensor glucose is >150 mg/dL and the correction bolus dose is calculated by the algorithm based on insulin requirement over the last 2–7 days. A temporary target that raises the sensor glucose target from the default of 126 mg/dL to 150 mg/dL may be used to mitigate exercise-induced hypoglycemia. CGM calibration is required at least every 12 h to remain in auto mode and bolus decisions require SMBG values, which are available via a Bluetooth-connected glucometer (Contour Next, Bayer).

Tandem t:slim X2 with Control-IQ works with the Dexcom G6 CGM system and the TypeZero control algorithm.[37] Control-IQ technology uses basal ICRs, and correction factors that are preset in the pump. In contrast to the 670G system, the present basal settings are incorporated into the algorithm and the system toggles between open loop and hybrid closed loop with little patient input required. Bolus and correctional doses administered by the users are delivered based on the CGM glucose values and calibration of the system or confirmation of BG values pre-bolus via SMBG is not required to remain in HCL. It similarly includes optional algorithm "tunings" for sleep and exercise activities. During sleep mode the system aims for a lower sensor glucose target by modulating basal insulin delivery, without delivering algorithm-directed correction boluses. During exercise mode the system is tuned to be less aggressive to allow for higher glucose targets (range 140–160 mg/dL) to mitigate exercise-induced hypoglycemia.

Future refinements in algorithm development and patient-centric advancements that allow for multiple inputs such as activity levels, as well as fully closed-loop versions that incorporate insulin only and dual hormonal insulin and glucagon or insulin and amylin delivery systems are under development.[38] Future systems are also likely to embed control functionality into consumer mobile device platforms once cybersecurity issues are addressed. In order for automated insulin delivery systems to reach their full potential, CGM accuracy and more rapidly absorbed insulin are core aspects that will need to be continuously refined.

CONCLUSION

Insulin pump therapy provides many advantages for patients with diabetes who are seeking improved glycemic control with less risk for hypoglycemia as well as increased lifestyle flexibility. More physiologic insulin delivery, less variability in insulin absorption, and several technical features that enable patients to modify insulin delivery according to their specific lifestyle preferences make insulin pump therapy an ideal treatment option for individuals seeking greater flexibility and more control over their diabetes self-management. Addition of CGM therapy can improve glycemic control and reduce risk of hypoglycemia independent of insulin administration methods. Integration of pump and CGM systems, or HCL systems, can further help patients to improve glycemic control using CGM metrics to modulate the amount of basal insulin administered and mitigate hypoglycemia, hyperglycemia and improve glycemic variability. The future is promising as improved technologies are applied to diabetes management.

REFERENCES

1. American Diabetes Association. 7. Diabetes technology: *Standards of Medical Care in Diabetes—2020*. *Diabetes Care* 2020;43(Suppl. 1):S77–S88

2. Pickup JC, Sutton AJ. Severe hypoglycaemia and glycaemic control in type 1 diabetes: meta-analysis of multiple daily insulin injections compared with continuous subcutaneous insulin infusion. *Diabetes Med* 2008;25(7):765–774

3. Riddell MC, Gallen IW, Smart CE, et al. Exercise management in type 1 diabetes: a consensus statement. *Lancet Diabetes Endocrinol* 2017;5(5):377–390

4. Lenhard MJ, Reeves GD. Continuous subcutaneous insulin infusion: a comprehensive review of insulin pump therapy. *Arch Intern Med* 2001;161(19): 2293–2300

5. Shetty G, Wolpert H. Insulin pump use in adults with type 1 diabetes—practical issues. *Diabetes Technol Ther* 2010;12(Suppl. 1):S11–S16

6. Bell KJ, Toschi E, Steil GM, Wolpert HA. Optimized mealtime insulin dosing for fat and protein in type 1 diabetes: application of a model-based approach to derive insulin doses for open-loop diabetes management. *Diabetes Care* 2016;39(9):1631–1634

7. Bell KJ, Fio CZ, Twigg S, et al. Amount and type of dietary fat, postprandial glycemia, and insulin requirements in type 1 diabetes: a randomized within-subject trial. *Diabetes Care* 2020;43(1):59–66

8. Bell KJ, Smart CE, Steil GM, et al. Impact of fat, protein, and glycemic index on postprandial glucose control in type 1 diabetes: implications for intensive diabetes management in the continuous glucose monitoring era. *Diabetes Care* 2015;38(6):1008–1015

9. Pasieka AM, Riddell MC. Advances in exercise, physical activity, and diabetes mellitus. *Diabetes Technol Ther* 2017;19(S1):S94–S104

10. Rigo RS, Levin LE, Belsito DV, et al. Cutaneous reactions to continuous glucose monitoring and continuous subcutaneous insulin infusion devices in type 1 diabetes mellitus. *J Diabetes Sci Technol* 2020;1932296820918894 [Epub ahead of print]

11. Umpierrez GE, Klonoff DC. Diabetes technology update: use of insulin pumps and continuous glucose monitoring in the hospital. *Diabetes Care* 2018;41(8):1579–1589

12. King BR, Goss PW, Paterson MA, Crock PA, Anderson DG. Changes in altitude cause unintended insulin delivery from insulin pumps: mechanisms and implications. *Diabetes Care* 2011;34(9):1932–1933

13. Wolpert HA, Faradji RN, Bonner-Weir S, Lipes MA. Metabolic decompensation in pump users due to lispro insulin precipitation. *BMJ* 2002; 324(7348):1253

14. Peters AL, Ahmann AJ, Battelino T, et al. Diabetes technology—continuous subcutaneous insulin infusion therapy and continuous glucose monitoring in adults: an Endocrine Society Clinical Practice Guideline. *J Clin Endocrinol Metab* 2016;101(11):3922–3937

15. Tamborlane WV, Beck RW, Bode BW, et al. Continuous glucose monitoring and intensive treatment of type 1 diabetes. *N Engl J Med* 2008;359(14): 1464–1476

16. Lind M, Polonsky W, Hirsch IB, et al. Continuous glucose monitoring vs conventional therapy for glycemic control in adults with type 1 diabetes treated with multiple daily insulin injections: the GOLD randomized clinical trial. *JAMA* 2017;317(4):379–387

17. Beck RW, Riddlesworth T, Ruedy K, et al. Effect of continuous glucose monitoring on glycemic control in adults with type 1 diabetes using insulin injections: the DIAMOND Randomized Clinical Trial. *JAMA* 2017;317(4): 371–378

18. Heinemann L, Freckmann G, Ehrmann D, et al. Real-time continuous glucose monitoring in adults with type 1 diabetes and impaired hypoglycaemia awareness or severe hypoglycaemia treated with multiple daily insulin injections (HypoDE): a multicentre, randomised controlled trial. *Lancet* 2018;391(10128):1367–1377

19. Polonsky WH, Hessler D, Ruedy KJ, Beck RW, DIAMOND Study Group. The impact of continuous glucose monitoring on markers of quality of life in adults with type 1 diabetes: further findings from the DIAMOND randomized clinical trial. *Diabetes Care* 2017;40(6):736–741

20. Beck RW, Riddlesworth TD, Ruedy K, et al. Continuous glucose monitoring versus usual care in patients with type 2 diabetes receiving multiple daily insulin injections: a randomized trial. *Ann Intern Med* 2017;167(6): 365–374

21. Feig DS, Donovan LE, Corcoy R, et al. Continuous glucose monitoring in pregnant women with type 1 diabetes (CONCEPTT): a multicentre international randomised controlled trial. *Lancet* 2017;390(10110):2347–2359

22. Kristensen K, Ögge LE, Sengpiel V, et al. Continuous Glucose glucose monitoring in pregnant women with type 1 diabetes: an observational cohort study of 186 pregnancies. *Diabetologia* 2019;62(7):1143–1153

23. Murphy HR, Rayman G, Duffield K, et al. Changes in the glycemic profiles of women with type 1 and type 2 diabetes during pregnancy. *Diabetes Care* 2007;30(11):2785–2791

24. Singh LG, Satyarengga M, Marcano I, et al. Reducing inpatient hypoglycemia in the general wards using real-time continuous glucose monitoring: The Glucose Telemetry System, a randomized clinical trial. *Diabetes Care* 2020;43(11):2736–2743

25. Shehav-Zaltzman G, Segal G, Konvalina N, Tirosh A. Remote glucose monitoring of hospitalized, quarantined patients with diabetes and COVID-19. *Diabetes Care* 2020;43(7):e75–e76

26. Ehrhardt N, Hirsch IB. The impact of COVID-19 on CGM use in the hospital. *Diabetes Care* 2020;43(11):2628–2630

27. Freckmann G, Schlüter S, Heinemann L, Diabetes Technology Working Group of the German Diabetes Society. Replacement of blood glucose measurements by measurements with systems for real-time continuous glucose

monitoring (rtCGM) or CGM with intermittent scanning (iscCGM): a German view. *J Diabetes Sci Technol* 2017;11(4):653–656

28. Edelman SV, Argento NB, Pettus J, Hirsch IB. Clinical implications of real-time and intermittently scanned continuous glucose monitoring. *Diabetes Care* 2018;41(11):2265–2274

29. Battelino T, Danne T, Bergenstal RM, et al. Clinical targets for continuous glucose monitoring data interpretation: recommendations from the International Consensus on Time in Range. *Diabetes Care* 2019;42(8):1593–1603

30. Vigersky RA, McMahon C. The relationship of hemoglobin A1C to time-in-range in patients with diabetes. *Diabetes Technol Ther* 2019;21(2):81–85

31. Bergenstal RM, Beck RW, Close KL, et al. Glucose management indicator (GMI): a new term for estimating A1C from continuous glucose monitoring. *Diabetes Care* 2018;41(11):2275–2280

32. Ceriello A, Monnier L, Owens D. Glycaemic variability in diabetes: clinical and therapeutic implications. *Lancet Diabetes Endocrinol* 2019;7(3):221–230

33. Johnson ML, Martens TW, Criego AB, et al. Utilizing the ambulatory glucose profile to standardize and implement continuous glucose monitoring in clinical practice. *Diabetes Technol Ther* 2019;21(S2):S217–S225

34. Aleppo G, Laffel LM, Ahmann AJ, et al. A practical approach to using trend arrows on the Dexcom G5 CGM system for the management of adults with diabetes. *J Endocr Soc* 2017;1(12):1445–1460

35. Leelarathna L, Choudhary P, Wilmot EG, et al. Hybrid closed-loop therapy: where are we in 2021? *Diabetes Obes Metab* 2021;23(3):655–660

36. Bergenstal RM, Garg S, Weinzimer SA, et al. Safety of a hybrid closed-loop insulin delivery system in patients with type 1 diabetes. *JAMA* 2016;316(13):1407–1408

37. Brown SA, Kovatchev BP, Raghinaru D, et al. Six-month randomized, multicenter trial of closed-loop control in type 1 diabetes. *N Engl J Med* 2019;381(18):1707–1717

38. Kesavadev J, Srinivasan S, Saboo B, Krishna BM, Krishnan G. The do-it-yourself artificial pancreas: a comprehensive review. *Diabetes Ther* 2020;11(6): 1217–1235

Monitoring

Highlights
Monitoring

■ Regular monitoring of blood glucose and diabetes-related laboratory testing is an essential component of any diabetes regimen. Frequency of monitoring can vary based on the patient's diabetes-related pharmacotherapy.

■ Glucose meters or continuous glucose monitoring allows for self-monitoring of blood glucose during intensive diabetes management.

■ Ketone monitoring by urine or blood can assist in monitoring for impending diabetic ketoacidosis.

■ Beyond routine monitoring of blood glucose, it is highly recommended to monitor blood glucose in the following scenarios: during symptoms of hypoglycemia, before operating an automobile, and before, during, and after exercise.

■ Advances in technology and electronic medical records have made it possible for the healthcare team to do remote glucose monitoring.

■ Monitoring of metabolic control and anthropometric measurements by the healthcare team at each visit should include
  • glycated hemoglobin A_{1c}—estimated 90-day average glucose,
  • review of blood glucose data and hypoglycemia events, and
  • assessment of growth, weight, and blood pressure.

■ Converting glycated hemoglobin A_{1c} measurements into an estimated average glucose value helps "translate" the glycated hemoglobin A_{1c} into a number patients can understand, and it makes treatment goals more understandable.

■ Monitoring the development and progression of long-term complications of diabetes should be performed at least as often as proposed by the American Diabetes Association in its Standards of Medical Care in Diabetes (see the section Monitoring for Long-Term Complications).

Monitoring

Regular monitoring by the patient and healthcare provider is an essential component of any diabetes management plan. Monitoring includes self-monitored blood glucose (SMBG) and ketone levels, assessment of metabolic control (diet, body mass index, laboratory evaluation), and screening for diabetes-related complications.

For the purposes of this chapter, intensive diabetes management is defined as basal-bolus insulin therapy consisting of at least three injections per day and frequent glucose monitoring. Glucose monitoring must be done more frequently than in less intensive diabetes management plans. This is true for both the medical monitoring performed by the healthcare team and the day-to-day monitoring required by the patient. Furthermore, monitoring by healthcare providers includes regular determination of hemoglobin A_{1c} (A1C), careful assessment of growth and development (in both children and adolescents) and weight (in adults), careful review of hypoglycemia episodes and related complications, review of ketone monitoring and sick-day management, and monitoring for the presence of diabetes-related complications.

MONITORING BY THE PATIENT

All patients using an intensive diabetes management program need to perform monitoring on a daily basis at home, work, school, or wherever they may be. Blood glucose monitoring can be performed using a glucose meter or a continuous glucose monitor (discussed in Chapter 7).

BLOOD GLUCOSE

In order to implement a successful intensive diabetes management plan consisting of basal-bolus therapy, patients should perform SMBG at least four times per day. Many patients often will perform SMBG four to six, or more, times a day. An inability or unwillingness to perform SMBG, or consistently wear a continuous glucose monitoring (CGM) device, should be considered a contraindication to implementing a basal-bolus insulin regimen. The addition of CGM can help decrease the burden of frequent fingersticks needed for SMBG and may provide the opportunity for intensive diabetes therapy in individuals who previously may not have been good candidates.[1]

The four essential SMBG determinations for successful implementation of a basal-bolus insulin therapy must be performed before each meal and before bedtime. Premeal measurements are needed to determine the dose of insulin, meal composition, or activity alterations required to achieve the target glucose level over the next few hours. These measurements also are used to determine patterns of glycemia over time that will guide adjustment of the regimen. It is best to observe these patterns over periods of at least 3–5 days before making an overall change in the regimen. The morning value is used to assess the adequacy of overnight glycemic control. The prelunch, predinner, and bedtime blood glucose measurements assess the adequacy of the mealtime dose of insulin for the meal prior to the reading. The bedtime blood glucose measurement is also a key safety component in allowing the opportunity for the patient to make insulin adjustments or eat a snack/meal in order to prevent nocturnal hypoglycemia.

In addition to these four blood glucose determinations, monitoring should include a periodic blood glucose measurement between 2:00 and 4:00 A.M. to detect unrecognized nocturnal hypoglycemia. This monitoring is especially important following more active days and for patients in whom the target blood glucose range is near the nondiabetic range or for patients in whom nocturnal or severe hypoglycemia or hypoglycemia unawareness has been a problem. Nocturnal monitoring may need to be performed more often than once a week during periods when the basal insulin dose is being adjusted. CGM provides a helpful way to monitor and alert the patient or caregiver to overnight hyper- or hypoglycemia and avoid unnecessarily waking the patient from sleep to perform a fingerstick.

Postprandial glycemia (PPG) contributes to overall blood glucose control and the A1C value.[2] Although the management of PPG can be challenging, it can be guided by attention to certain behaviors and pharmacological therapy. These interventions include monitoring PPG by fingerstick or CGM to provide insight into methods to lower elevated PPG. Some methods to lower PPG include adjusting the premeal insulin dose; injecting rapid-acting insulin analogs 15–20 min before eating; doing 10–20 min of moderate exercise within 1 h of eating; delaying the intake of carbohydrates from the meal to allow insulin to start working, when a bolus 15–20 min before the meal is not possible; and utilizing ultra-rapid-acting insulin analogs or Technosphere inhaled insulin. Although patients may report improvement in quality-of-life measures with improved postprandial glycemia control, the impact of postprandial hyperglycemia on diabetes-related complications is unclear. The strongest established relationship is postprandial hyperglycemia in pregnancy and the development of macrosomia, but studies outside of pregnancy suggest associations between postprandial hyperglycemia and diabetic retinopathy and cardiovascular disease. Further studies are ongoing to examine the relationship between postprandial glycemia and longer-term outcomes.

Monitoring blood glucose when symptoms of hypoglycemia occur is strongly recommended. Because hypoglycemia can occur with few or no early warning symptoms (hypoglycemia unawareness), and because autonomic (adrenergic) symptoms can occur in the absence of hypoglycemia, patients should confirm biochemical hypoglycemia by measuring their blood glucose level when symptoms occur.

Because driving ability may be impaired at blood glucose levels higher than those that usually trigger easily recognizable hypoglycemia symptoms (especially in patients with hypoglycemia unawareness and those using basal-bolus therapy), it is strongly recommended that blood glucose be monitored before driving.

Blood glucose can drop more rapidly during strenuous physical activity or exercise. Therefore, blood glucose should be monitored before, during, and after activity. Insulin adjustments may need to be made before and after activity.[3] Some patients may find it helpful to take less insulin (e.g., 50% less) if they plan to exercise within 3–4 h of an insulin bolus.

CGM should be strongly considered for all patients using intensive diabetes management and should be regarded as being part of the standard of care for individuals with type 1 diabetes (T1D).[4] A continuous glucose monitor is helpful in decreasing the burden of SMBG; providing pre- and postmeal glucose assessments; alerting to real-time, impending, and retrospective hypoglycemic events; and allowing for glucose monitoring when fingersticks would otherwise be difficult or inconvenient (e.g., while driving or exercising; see Chapter 7 for more detail).

KETONE MONITORING

Monitoring for the presence of ketones is an essential component of diabetes care. In certain situations, ketone monitoring is necessary for the safe implementation of diabetes therapy, regardless of the type of therapy used (see Table 8.1).

Ketone monitoring can be done using strips that measure urine ketones (acetoacetate and acetone) or with a specific meter that measures blood β-hydroxybutyrate (BHB) concentration. This device is similar to other SMBG meters and also can measure blood glucose levels using a different strip in the same meter. The advantages of urine monitoring strips include ease of sample collection under most circumstances and low cost. Measurement of blood ketones offers the

Table 8.1—Patient Monitoring during Intensive Diabetes Management

- Self-monitoring of blood glucose
  - Before each meal
  - At bedtime
  - Between 2:00 and 4:00 A.M., when deemed relevant by healthcare provider
  - When symptoms of hypoglycemia occur
  - Before driving
  - Before, during, and after exercise and increased physical activity
- Ketone monitoring
  - During illness
  - During unexpected or persistent hyperglycemia
  - With nausea, vomiting, abdominal pain
  - For patients on sodium–glucose cotransporter 2 (SGLT2) inhibitors: symptoms such as nausea that could be indicative of ketosis

Of note: SGLT2 inhibitors are not approved by the U.S. Food and Drug Administration for the treatment of T1D.

special advantage in young children who may not be able to provide a urine sample on demand for urine ketone testing, especially during illness. Under these circumstances, measurement of blood ketone levels may prevent a trip to the emergency department. Blood ketone determination is significantly more expensive than urine ketone determination, but in some circumstances it may be cost-effective.

Blood or urine ketones should be checked whenever the blood glucose level is unexpectedly or repeatedly >250–300 mg/dL (>13.8–16.7 mmol/L). The same is true during intercurrent illness, especially a gastrointestinal illness, regardless of the blood glucose concentration. Illness can trigger diabetic ketoacidosis (DKA), thus, rapid identification and intervention can prevent severe illness and possible hospitalization. In addition, ketosis can cause nausea, vomiting, and abdominal pain. Of note, euglycemic DKA has been reported in patients using sodium–glucose cotransporter 2 (SGLT2) inhibitors. This includes patients with type 2 diabetes (T2D) and patients with T1D using these agents off-label.[5] Therefore, patients on SGLT2 inhibitors need to be aware of the potential risk of DKA development. For patients with T2D, those with long-standing T2D with marked β-cell insufficiency or evolving latent autoimmune diabetes appear to be at higher risk. These patients should be counseled to check ketones in the case of prolonged starvation, after surgery, during an acute illness, or when experiencing symptoms of unexplained nausea and vomiting.[6]

For patients using an insulin pump, ketones should be measured whenever they experience unexplained hyperglycemia (≥250 mg/dL before breakfast or persistent blood glucose levels >250 mg/dL during the day). In this setting, the presence of ketonuria or ketonemia may indicate failure of the insulin delivery system. Moderate to "large" ketone readings using urine acetoacetate measurement strips (Ketostix, Bayer) may indicate impending or overt ketoacidosis. Ketone strips are widely available in pharmacies, relatively cheap in comparison to blood ketone measurement, and may not require a prescription. However, they are less accurate than blood ketone measurement, providing only a semiquantitive measure of acetoacetate, and can be affected by kidney function and hydration status. Blood ketone meters are also available and measure BHB, a more accurate measure of real-time ketogenesis. However, blood ketone strips are more expensive than urinary ketone strips and may not be covered by some health insurances. Normal BHB concentrations are <0.6 mmol/L. Concentrations >3 mmol/L are suggestive of ketoacidosis in the appropriate clinical setting. Urinary ketones should be monitored daily in women who are pregnant.

MONITORING BY THE HEALTHCARE TEAM

Overall metabolic control in people with diabetes is assessed primarily by five factors:

- SMBG
- Average blood glucose and A1C levels
- Frequency and severity of hypoglycemia
- Adequacy of growth, weight gain, and physical development in children and weight in adults
- Plasma lipid levels

Table 8.2—Monitoring Metabolic Control

- Routinely determine A1C (estimated average glucose)
- Review SMBG results carefully at every visit as well as between visits (if necessary)
- Review the frequency, severity, recognition, and treatment of hypoglycemia
- Assess growth, weight gain, and physical development in children and adolescents and weight in adults
- Take a careful history related to the management of sick days and occurrence of ketoacidosis
- Review issues of diet, including weight, and any difficulties in adherence to the overall management plan
- Monitor blood lipids annually

At the outset of intensive diabetes management, after daily to weekly office visits when the program is being implemented and adjusted, the patient will require scheduled visits to assess the success of the program (see Table 8.2).

It is common practice to assess a patient's glycemic control and general health status quarterly. This schedule usually is sufficient for the patient using intensive diabetes management after the initial phase of stabilization. At each visit

- measure A1C;
- check accuracy of blood glucose monitoring;
- review blood glucose data;
- study problems with hypoglycemia;
- identify and discuss any barriers to intensive diabetes management;
- discuss issues of diet;
- note body weight, blood pressure, and growth and physical development in children; and
- examine sites of insulin administration.

A1C—ESTIMATED AVERAGE GLUCOSE

The A1C test reflects mean glycemia over the preceding 3 months and is an essential component of diabetes management. A1C should be measured at least twice a year in patients who are meeting treatment goals and quarterly in patients whose therapy has changed or who are not at goal. More frequent A1C measurements may be useful during periods of changing diabetes management. Converting A1C measurements into an estimated average glucose value translates the A1C into a number that patients can understand more readily and may make treatment goals more intelligible (see Table 8.3). Individual variations in the rate of hemoglobin glycation, however, can contribute to inaccuracy in estimating the average glucose from A1C levels, and it is important for clinicians to inform patients about this uncertainty[7] (see Table 8.4).

Notably, there are conditions associated with an altered relationship between A1C and glycemia. Hemoglobin variants, such as sickle-cell disease, can interfere with the measurement of A1C, although most assays in the U.S. are unaffected by the most common hemoglobin variants. Other conditions that could alter the A1C result are

Table 8.3 — Correlation between A1C Level and Estimated Average Glucose Level

A1C (%)	Glucose level	
	mg/dL (95% CI)	mmol/L
6	126 (100–152)	7.0 (5.5–8.5)
7	154 (123–185)	8.6 (6.8–10.3)
8	183 (147–217)	10.2 (8.1–12.1)
9	212 (170–249)	11.8 (9.4–13.9)
10	240 (193–282)	13.4 (10.7–15.7)
11	269 (217–314)	14.9 (12.0–17.5)
12	298 (240–347)	16.5 (13.3–19.3)

pregnancy, glucose-6-phosphate dehydrogenase deficiency, hemodialysis, recent blood loss or transfusion, or erythropoietin therapy. A1C is also less reliable in conditions such as the postpartum state, patients with HIV treated with certain drugs, and iron deficiency anemia. In cases where the A1C is unreliable, the examination of SMBG measurements and use of the ambulatory glucose profile (AGP) and/or other CGM-derived metrics are useful to determine the degree of glycemic control.[8]

With the development of highly accurate CGM technologies, physicians and patients can now reliably use these data for glucose monitoring and treatment decisions. CGM data for at least 10–14 days provides sufficient data to represent a mean glucose value called the glucose management indicator (GMI). GMI is estimated from a formula derived from a plot of CGM-measured mean glucose concentration versus central laboratory-measured A1C (GMI [%] = 3.31 + 0.02392 × [mean glucose in mg/dL] or GMI (mmol/mol) = 12.71 + 4.70587 × [mean glucose in mmol/L] (Table 8.5).

A calculator to compute GMI is available. The GMI in combination with the measured A1C value can guide the provider in glucose management. Further-

Table 8.4 — Causes of Falsely Low or High A1C Levels

Falsely low A1C	Falsely high A1C
Hemolysis	Iron deficiency anemia
Post-treatment of iron/B12/folate deficiency anemia	Uremia
Red blood cell transfusion	Alcoholism
Acute blood loss	B12 deficiency anemia
Chronic liver disease	Folate deficiency anemia
Erythropoietin treatment	

Table 8.5—GMI Calculated for Various CGM-Derived Mean Glucose Concentrations

CGM-derived mean glucose (mg/dL)	GMI (%)
100	5.7
125	6.3
150	6.9
175	7.5
200	8.1
225	8.7
250	9.3
275	9.9
300	10.5
350	11.7
CGM-measured mean glucose (mmol/L)	**GMI (mmol/mol)**
5	36.2
6	40.9
7	45.7
8	50.4
9	55.1
10	59.8
12	69.2
14	78.6
16	88.0
18	97.4

Source—Adapted from Bergenstal.[8]

more, the GMI can give patients and providers a perspective on where the overall laboratory A1C is trending in a shorter time window to know if treatment modifications are having an impact.

Point-of-care (POC) A1C testing devices are increasingly available for use during outpatient visits, using a bench-top analyzer and fingerstick blood samples.[9] Although POC A1C testing should ideally not be used for the purposes of diagnosing diabetes, given slight variation in precision as compared to the reference laboratory standard, it can be useful for POC monitoring in patients with known diabetes where small degrees of variation are less likely to change therapy decisions.[10] For more detailed discussion of the value of CGM technology, please review Chapter 7.

The long-term complications of diabetes include retinopathy and cataracts, renal insufficiency and hypertension, autonomic and peripheral neuropathy, and macrovascular disease manifested by myocardial infarction, stroke, and peripheral vascular disease. Although improved glycemic control with intensive diabetes therapy delays the onset and slows the progression of retinopathy, nephropathy, and neuropathy and improves the risk factor profile related to macrovascular disease, complications of diabetes have not yet been eliminated. Therefore, monitoring for their presence and appropriate intervention or referral to appropriate specialists are required (see Table 8.6).

RETINAL EXAMINATIONS

A comprehensive examination by an optometrist or ophthalmologist is recommended for all patients with T2D at the time of diagnosis, for all patients with T1D within 5 years after diagnosis, and for any patient with diabetes who has visual symptoms or abnormalities. Subsequent examinations should be repeated at least annually, or more frequently if advanced retinopathy is noted. If there is no evidence of retinopathy for one or more annual eye exams and glycemia is well controlled, then screening every 2 years may be considered. Women with preexisting T1D or T2D who are planning pregnancy or who are pregnant should have a comprehensive eye examination before pregnancy or during the first trimester, and then monitored every trimester and for 1 year postpartum as indicated by the degree of retinopathy.[11]

Table 8.6—Monitoring for Long-Term Complications

- Comprehensive annual dilated eye and visual examination, beginning when diagnosed with T2D, at a duration of T1D of 5 years, or when any visual symptoms of abnormalities occur
  - Frequency of comprehensive dilated eye exams can be reduced to every 2 years per the treating physician's discretion if there is no evidence of retinopathy.
- Screening blood lipids at diagnosis and then every 5 years if under age 40, or more frequently if indicated
- Careful examination of the feet (history, skin inspection, pinprick sensation, vibration sensation, dorsalis pedis and posterior tibial artery pulses, deep tendon reflexes) at least annually
  - Patients with evidence of sensory loss should have feet inspected at every visit.
- Careful assessment of blood pressure at each visit
- Annual determination of urinary albumin (e.g., spot urinary albumin-to-creatinine ratio) and estimated glomerular filtration rate should be assessed in patients with T1D with duration of ≥5 years and in all patients with T2D.
- Patients with diabetes and urinary albumin >300 mg/g creatinine and/or an estimated glomerular filtration rate 30–60 mL/min/1.73 m^2 should be monitored twice annually to guide therapy.

Retinopathy initially may worsen during the first months of intensive diabetes management. This worsening is more often reported in patients who have poor glycemic control and more advanced retinopathy before the initiation of intensive therapy. In the Diabetes Control and Complications Trial (DCCT), retinopathy progression was greater in the intensively treated cohort at the end of the first year. By the end of the second year, this difference was not significant, and thereafter the intensively treated cohort had a lower rate of retinopathy progression. Therefore, any patients undertaking intensive management should have a retinal examination before beginning intensive management and should discuss the plans for intensive management with their eye care professional, especially if metabolic control has been poor.

LIPID SCREENING

Lipid abnormalities play an important role in macrovascular disease. In recognition of this, diabetes is regarded as a risk factor for cardiovascular events equivalent to a previous cardiac event. In adults, a screening lipid profile should be performed at the time of first diagnosis, at the initial medical evaluation, or at age 40 years and periodically (e.g., every 1–2 years) thereafter. A lipid panel should be obtained immediately before initiating statin therapy and then 4–12 weeks following initiation to assess medical adherence, liver enzymes, and efficacy. Once therapy and response are stable, a once-yearly lipid panel can be obtained to confirm continued efficacy and adherence.[12]

In contrast to former recommendations targeting specific LDL levels for primary prevention, statin therapy should be initiated based on cardiovascular disease risk in diabetes. Beneficial effects have been reported in people with diabetes with and without coronary heart disease. Patients aged 40–75 years should be on moderate-intensity statin therapy if they have no additional atherosclerotic cardiovascular disease (ASCVD) risk factors. If they have additional ASCVD risk factors (e.g., dyslipidemia, hypertension, smoking, obesity), their ASCVD risk is ≥20%, or they are aged 50–70 years, high-intensity statins should be considered (Table 8.7).

Table 8.7 — High-Intensity and Moderate-Intensity Statin Therapy

High-intensity statin therapy (lowers LDL cholesterol by ≥50%)	Moderate-intensity statin therapy (lowers LDL cholesterol by 30–49%)
Atorvastatin 40–80 mg	Atorvastatin 10–20 mg
Rosuvastatin 20–40 mg	Rosuvastatin 5–10 mg
	Simvastatin 20–40 mg
	Pravastatin 40–80 mg
	Lovastatin 40 mg
	Fluvastatin XL 80 mg
	Pitavastatin 1–4 mg

Source—Adapted from American Diabetes Association.[12]

(The ASCVD risk assessment tool is available online at tools.acc.org/ASCVD -Risk-Estimator-Plus.) Of note, recommendations for people with T1D are mostly extrapolated from interventional trials in adults with T2D. Adults with T1D who have abnormal lipids and additional risk factors for ASCVD should be treated with statins.[13] All adults with diabetes who have known ASCVD should be treated with statins, regardless of additional risk factors, for secondary prevention.[12]

BLOOD PRESSURE

Hypertension is major risk factor for both ASCVD and microvascular complications. Numerous studies have reported that antihypertensive therapy reduces ASCVD events, heart failure, and microvascular complications. Therefore, blood pressure should be measured at every routine clinical visit. If the blood pressure is ≥140/90 mmHg at a visit, it needs to be confirmed on a separate day prior to diagnosis of hypertension. Once the diagnosis of hypertension is established, patients with diabetes should monitor their blood pressure at least weekly at home and alert their provider if they are noting blood pressure above the therapeutic target.

Blood pressure therapeutic targets differ based on underlying risk factors and are frequently reviewed and updated by various professional societies and guideline writing groups. In general, for individuals with diabetes and hypertension at lower risk of ASCVD, treating to a blood pressure target of <140/90 mmHg is reasonable. For individuals with diabetes and risk factors for ASCVD or a 10-year ASCVD risk ≥15%, then a target of <130/80 would be appropriate if tolerated. Treatment for hypertension should include drug classes such as ACE inhibitors, angiotensin receptor blockers, thiazide-like diuretics, or dihydropyridine calcium channel blockers that may reduce cardiovascular events in people with diabetes. ACE inhibitors or angiotensin receptor blockers are preferred in people who have hypertenstion and albuminuria.[12]

URINARY ALBUMIN SCREENING

Measurement of urinary albumin excretion should be performed annually in all individuals ≥10 years old with T1D duration of at least 5 years. Because of the difficulty in precisely dating the onset of T2D, such screening should begin at the time of diagnosis in adults and in children and adolescents with T2D. Screening for albuminuria can be performed by measuring the albumin-to-creatinine ratio in a random, spot urine collection. Screening may be confounded by orthostatic proteinuria; therefore, abnormal results should indicate repeated screening. A diagnosis of albuminuria can be made based on abnormal first morning urine specimens two to three times within a 3- to 6-month period. Exercise within 24 h, infection, fever, congestive heart failure, marked hyperglycemia, menstruation, and marked hypertension may elevated the urine albumin-to-creatinine ratio independent of kidney damage.[14]

FOOT EXAMINATIONS

Patients should have an annual foot examination to identify high-risk foot conditions related to diabetes. The examination should include inspection to assess hygiene and to determine the presence of any ulcers or infection. The assessment also should include a careful history to ascertain the presence of numbness, paresthesiae (tingling), or weakness. Posterior tibial and dorsalis pedis pulses should be palpated, and deep tendon ankle reflexes and sensation should be checked. Individuals who have reduced sensation or pulses, foot deformities, or callus formation should have a careful foot examination at each routine office visit.[14]

REFERENCES

1. Halbron M, Bourron O, Andreelli F, et al. Insulin pump combined with flash glucose monitoring: a therapeutic option to improve glycemic control in severely nonadherent patients with type 1 diabetes. *Diabetes Technol Ther* 2019;21(7):409–412

2. Leahy JJL, Aleppo G, Fonseca VA, et al. Optimizing postprandial glucose management in adults with insulin-requiring diabetes: report and recommendations. *J Endocr Soc* 2019;3(10):1942–1957

3. Riddell MC, Gallen IW, Smart CE, et al. Exercise management in type 1 diabetes: a consensus statement. *Lancet Diabetes Endocrinol* 2017;5(5): 377–390

4. American Diabetes Association. 7. Diabetes technology: *Standards of Medical Care in Diabetes—2020. Diabetes Care* 2020;43(Suppl. 1):S77–S88

5. Rosenstock J, Ferrannini E. Euglycemic diabetic ketoacidosis: a predictable, detectable, and preventable safety concern with SGLT2 inhibitors. *Diabetes Care* 2015;38(9):1638–1642

6. Liu J, Li L, Li S, et al. Sodium-glucose co-transporter-2 inhibitors and the risk of diabetic ketoacidosis in patients with type 2 diabetes: a systematic review and meta-analysis of randomized controlled trials. *Diabetes Obes Metab* 2020;22(9):1619–1627

7. Radin MS. Pitfalls in hemoglobin A1c measurement: when results may be misleading. *J Gen Intern Med* 2014;29(2):388–394

8. Bergenstal RM, Beck RW, Close KL, et al. Glucose management indicator (GMI): a new term for estimating A1C from continuous glucose monitoring. *Diabetes Care* 2018;41(11):2275–2280

9. O'Brien MJ, Sacks DB. Point-of-care hemoglobin A1c. *JAMA* 2019;322(14): 1404–1405

10. Nathan DM, Griffin A, Perez FM, et al. Accuracy of a point-of-care hemoglobin A1c assay. *J Diabetes Sci Technol* 2019;13(6):1149–1153

11. American Diabetes Association. 14. Management of diabetes in pregnancy: *Standards of Medical Care in Diabetes—2020. Diabetes Care* 2020;43(Suppl. 1): S183–S192

12. American Diabetes Association. 10. Cardiovascular disease and risk management: *Standards of Medical Care in Diabetes—2020*. *Diabetes Care* 2020; 43(Suppl. 1):S111–S134

13. de Ferranti SD, de Boer IH, Fonseca V, et al. Type 1 diabetes mellitus and cardiovascular disease: a scientific statement from the American Heart Association and American Diabetes Association. *Diabetes Care* 2014;37(10): 2843–2863

14. American Diabetes Association. 11. Microvascular complications and foot care: *Standards of Medical Care in Diabetes—2020*. *Diabetes Care* 2020;43(Suppl. 1): S135–S151

Nutrition Management

Highlights
Nutrition Management

- Medical nutrition therapy is integral to the implementation of all forms of intensified diabetes care.

- The primary goals of medical nutrition therapy are to promote healthy eating by focusing on nutrient-dense foods and portion sizes in order to improve metabolic status, including glycated hemoglobin A_{1c}, blood pressure, and lipid levels. The nutrition plan must also prevent, or at least slow, the development of long-term diabetes complications, address individual nutrition needs (taking into account personal preferences, willingness to change, and economic considerations), and promote pleasurable eating.

- Medical nutrition therapy is often the most challenging aspect of diabetes management, leading to the recommendation that every person with diabetes should regularly consult a registered dietitian nutritionist knowledgeable about diabetes for development and periodic reevaluation of a personalized meal plan. Outcome studies demonstrate that medical nutrition therapy provided by registered dietitian nutritionists can result in up to 2.0% reduction in glycated hemoglobin A_{1c} in type 2 diabetes, and up to a 1.9% reduction in type 1 diabetes at 3–6 months.

- Target nutrition recommendations:
  - Urge development of a personalized plan based on an individual assessment,
  - Emphasize total carbohydrate intake as the primary nutrition factor affecting postprandial blood glucose levels, but also consider the type of carbohydrate ingested and the fat and protein content of the meal,
  - Emphasize the role of weight loss in type 2 diabetes as a strategy to decrease insulin resistance and achieve glycemic and metabolic control.

- In type 1 diabetes, the meal plan should be based on the patient's usual intake with respect to calories, food selection, and meal timing. The insulin regimen should be complementary to the meal plan and adjusted based on the results of glucose monitoring.

- In type 2 diabetes, the dietitian should review the patient's usual intake and advise the patient to distribute calories and carbohydrates throughout the day, avoiding large concentrations at any one time. If the patient is overweight or obese, a healthy eating plan with an energy deficit for weight loss should be recommended, in concert with advice regarding physical activity and other behavioral or lifestyle modifications, as needed.

- Carbohydrate counting is a meal-planning approach well suited to intensive diabetes management because it allows matching of mealtime insulin delivery to carbohydrate-related insulin requirement.
- Glucose monitoring is an essential component of all approaches to intensive diabetes management. The joint evaluation of food and glucose records is an important tool for glucose control and allows fine-tuning of both nutrition and medication treatment plans.
- Hypoglycemia is a significant risk of intensive management. Nutrition factors often play a role in the cause and prevention of hypoglycemia.
- Avoidance of hyperglycemia and greater precision in glucose control can be achieved through calibrated treatment of hypoglycemia, taking into account both the patient's dose response to oral glucose and the current and target glucose values.
- Weight gain may accompany intensive management when significant improvement in glucose control is achieved and is related to a reduction of glycosuria and consumption of extra calories to treat more frequent hypoglycemia. Strategies to prevent weight gain include reducing calories at the outset of intensive management, increasing physical activity, and rigorous medical nutrtion therapy.

Nutrition Management

Medical nutrition therapy (MNT) is integral to successful diabetes management and is especially important for intensive diabetes management. Patients who use basal-bolus insulin regimens and perform frequent capillary blood glucose measurements or use continuous glucose monitoring (CGM) to maintain tight glucose control must apply sophisticated nutrition management skills to fully realize the potential of their intensive management plan. As demonstrated in the Diabetes Control and Complications Trial (DCCT), extensive, individualized nutrition training and problem-solving are required to support effective intensive management in patients with type 1 diabetes (T1D).[1]

MNT is recommended for all individuals with both T1D and type 2 diabetes (T2D) at the time of diagnosis and for ongoing follow-up. Unfortunately, only about half of all patients will receive nutrition education and far less will receive intensive nutrition management.[2] Insulin initiation appears to be the most common factor that triggers primary care physicians to refer patients with T2D for nutrition counseling. Those patients who manage their diabetes with lifestyle modification or oral hypoglycemic agents or for whom nutrition is the primary or sole treatment modality are least likely to receive assistance with the nutrition component of their management. Extending MNT to this population would, in itself, represent a major "intensification" of their care.

GOALS OF MEDICAL NUTRITION THERAPY

The overall goal of MNT in diabetes care is to promote healthy eating patterns. Included in this general objective are several specific targets (see Table 9.1). To achieve these goals, dietitians and other healthcare professionals must educate people with diabetes to manage their nutrition intake with respect to a variety of individual factors, including medication, physical activity, illness and other stressors, and lifestyle considerations (e.g., work or school schedules, personal preferences, motivation, and economic, cultural, and religious concerns).

Consistent management and modification of food intake are often the most complex and challenging aspects of diabetes care. The complexity of these tasks is due to many factors (see Table 9.2). For this reason, every person with prediabetes or diabetes should consult a registered dietitian nutritionist (RD/RDN), preferably one familiar with the components of diabetes MNT, to obtain an individual nutrition plan. Because nutrition intake interacts with medication and physical

Table 9.1—Goals of MNT Applicable to All Individuals with Diabetes

- Promote and support healthful eating patterns, emphasizing a variety of nutrient-dense foods in appropriate portion sizes, to improve overall health and
  - Achieve and maintain body weight
  - Attain individualized glycemic, blood pressure, and lipid goals
  - Delay or prevent the complications of diabetes
- Address individual nutrition needs, taking into account personal and cultural preferences; health literacy; food security; access to healthy food choices; readiness, willingness, and ability to change; and barriers to change.
- Promote pleasurable eating by providing nonjudgmental messages about food choices while modifying food choices only if indicated by scientific evidence.
- Provide practical tools for individuals with diabetes for developing healthy eating patterns rather than focusing on individual macronutrients, micronutrients, or single foods.

activity in determining blood glucose levels, nutrition care must be fully integrated with other aspects of diabetes management to be effective. This is best accomplished through a team approach. At a minimum, however, successful MNT requires open communication between the dietitian and other care providers. Furthermore, patients will likely benefit most from a series of encounters dedicated to nutrition education and problem-solving to help develop the sophisticated skills required for successful management. Regular review and adjustment of the nutrition plan are also needed for optimal results.[2]

TARGET NUTRITION RECOMMENDATIONS

The current nutrition principles and recommendations for diabetes, as formulated by the American Diabetes Association, focus on lifestyle goals and strategies for both the prevention and treatment of diabetes (see Table 9.3).

Table 9.2—Factors That Contribute to the Complexity of Nutrition Care

- Interaction of diabetes MNT with coexisting pathology (e.g., abnormal lipids, elevated blood pressure, and other health problems)
- Need to integrate MNT into other components of diabetes treatment regimen
- Need for advanced problem-solving skills to permit self-management
- Need for stepwise training to progressively build requisite knowledge and skills
- Inherent difficulty in modifying lifelong food behaviors and preferences
- Dynamic nature of both diabetes and life circumstances that demands periodic and creative modification of nutrition plan
- Need to meet all of these challenges while preserving patient autonomy and quality of life

Table 9.3—Target Nutrition Recommendations for All People with Diabetes

Carbohydrate

- A dietary pattern that includes carbohydrate from fruits, vegetables, whole grains, legumes, and dairy products is encouraged for good health.
- Monitoring carbohydrate, whether by carbohydrate counting, or experience-based estimation, is a key strategy in achieving glycemic control.
- There is some evidence that lower-carbohydrate diets can be effective to improve glycemic control; however, the amount of carbohydrate has not been defined and the long-term sustainability of low-carbohydrate diets has been a challenge for many.[2]
- The use of the glycemic index and glycemic load may modestly improve glycemic control (at least when compared with considering total carbohydrate alone).[3]
- Sucrose-containing foods can be substituted for other carbohydrates in the meal plan or, if added to the meal plan, can be covered with insulin or other glucose-lowering medications. Care should be taken to avoid excess energy intake and maintain nutritional balance.
- Sugar alcohols and nonnutritive sweeteners are safe when consumed within the daily intake levels established by the U.S. Food and Drug Administration (FDA) and appear to have minimal glycemic effect.[2] Nonnutritive sweeteners may be a reasonable short-term substitute for sugar. However, decreased consumption of both sugar and nonnutritive sweeteners should be encouraged.
- People with diabetes are encouraged to consume a variety of fiber-containing foods, especially from vegetables, legumes, fruits, and whole grains. Increasing fiber intake above the recommendations for the general public may modestly lower glycated hemoglobin A_{1c} (A1C).[2]

Protein

- For individuals with diabetes and normal renal function, evidence is insufficient to suggest that standard protein intake recommendations (15–20% of energy) should be modified.
- In individuals with T2D, ingested protein can increase insulin response without increasing plasma glucose concentrations. Therefore, protein should not be used to treat acute hypoglycemia or to prevent nighttime hypoglycemia.
- In individuals with T1D, ingested protein can increase blood glucose concentrations in the absence of sufficient active insulin. Individuals observing such an effect of dietary protein may benefit from education and adjustment of prandial insulin doses accordingly.
- The long-term effects of protein intake >20% of calories on diabetes management are unknown. Although such diets may produce short-term weight loss and improve glycemia, it has not been established that these benefits are maintained, and long-term effects on kidney function for people with diabetes are unknown.[2]

Fat

- Evidence is inconclusive for an ideal amount of total fat intake for people with diabetes; therefore, goals should be individualized. Fat quality appears to be far more important than quantity.
  - In people with T2D, a Mediterranean-style diet, following a monounsaturated fatty acid–rich eating pattern, may be beneficial to glycemic control and may reduce risk factors for cardiovascular disease. This eating pattern may be an effective alternative to a lower-fat, higher-carbohydrate eating pattern.
  - Evidence does not support recommending omega-3 (EPA and DHA) supplements for people with diabetes for the prevention or treatment of cardiovascular events.

- As recommended for the general public, an increase in foods containing long-chain omega-3 fatty acids (EPA and DHA) from fatty fish and omega-3 linolenic acid (ALA) is recommended for individuals with diabetes because of their beneficial effects on lipoproteins, prevention of heart disease, and associations with positive health outcomes in observational studies.[4]
- The recommendation for the general public to eat fish (particularly fatty fish) at least two times (two servings) per week is also appropriate for people with diabetes.
- The amount of dietary saturated fat, cholesterol, and trans fat recommended for people with diabetes is the same as that recommended for the general population.
- In individuals with T1D, dietary fat can indirectly increase blood glucose concentrations in the absence of sufficient active insulin, primarily through increased acute insulin resistance and hepatic glucose output. Individuals observing such an effect of dietary fat may benefit from education and adjustment of prandial insulin doses accordingly.[2]

Macronutrients

- Despite numerous studies, the optimal macronutrient composition for diabetes management has not been identified. Therefore, meals should be individualized for metabolic goals, physical activity, and food preferences.[2]

Micronutrients

- There is no clear evidence of a benefit from vitamin or mineral supplementation in people with diabetes who do not have underlying deficiencies compared with the general population.
- Individual meal planning should include optimization of food choices to meet recommended daily allowance/dietary reference intake for all micronutrients.
- Routine supplementation of chromium, vitamin D, or herbal supplements (including cinnamon, curcumin, or aloe vera) has not been clearly demonstrated and therefore cannot be recommended.[2]
- There is recent evidence that individuals taking metformin are at a higher risk for vitamin B12 deficiency (especially those with anemia or peripheral neuropathy), and laboratory evaluation of vitamin B12 status should be considered.[2]

Alcohol

- If adults with diabetes choose to consume alcohol, daily intake should be limited to a moderate amount (one drink per day or less for adult women and two drinks per day or less for adult men). One drink is defined as 12 oz beer, 5 oz wine, or 1.5 oz ~80-proof spirits.
- Alcohol acutely impairs glucose release from the liver. To reduce the risk of hypoglycemia in individuals using insulin or insulin secretagogues, alcohol should be consumed with food and blood glucose levels monitored closely for 12–24 h.
- In individuals with diabetes, moderate consumption of alcohol may have a minimal effect on glucose and insulin concentrations, but when combined in carbohydrate-containing beverages—such as mixed drinks, sweet wines, and regular beer—it may raise blood glucose.[2]

A personalized nutrition prescription should be based on individual assessment and should consider treatment goals and lifestyle changes the patient is willing and able to make. Clinical outcomes should be monitored and, if necessary, the nutrition prescription should be modified. This method has replaced specific guidelines for one "standard" diet or meal planning method for all people with diabetes.[5]

The recommendations acknowledge scientific evidence that sucrose and other simple sugars do not inherently impair diabetes control, opening the way for the inclusion of many traditionally "forbidden" foods in diabetes meal plans.

Modest weight loss (5% body weight) decreases insulin resistance in individuals with diabetes who are overweight or obese. Weight loss of 15% has been reported to provide optimal outcomes for glycemic control in patients with T2D and weight loss of 7–10% significantly decreases the risk of developing T2D in patients with prediabetes.[2] The overarching goal for people with diabetes is to achieve blood glucose, blood pressure, and blood lipid levels in the normal range, or as close to normal as is safely possible, whether by weight loss or other means. Standardized diets and simplistic advice to "avoid sugar" and "lose weight," which have too often accounted for the totality of nutrition advice, are clearly inadequate. The current guidelines are compatible with a shift to more intensive programs of management for all people with diabetes. A flowchart describing the major steps in the design and implementation of meal plans consistent with the current recommendations is shown in Fig. 9.1.[2] Some ways to integrate recommendations into the nutrition care process are listed in Table 9.4.

STRATEGIES FOR TYPE 1 DIABETES

The following strategies are the starting points for the MNT component of intensified management for people with T1D. They form the basis of care, regardless of the specific meal-planning approach used.

- Insulin therapy should be integrated into an individual's dietary and physical activity pattern.
- Individuals using rapid-acting insulin, either by injection or insulin pump, should adjust meal and snack insulin doses based on the amount of carbohydrate in their meals and snacks.
- Individuals using fixed daily insulin doses should keep daily carbohydrate intake consistent with respect to time and amount.
- For planned exercise, insulin doses can be adjusted. For unplanned exercise, extra carbohydrate may be needed.

Maintaining a consistent carbohydrate intake can be extremely challenging. On presentation, newly diagnosed individuals with T1D often have experienced weight loss and have an increase in appetite with the initiation of insulin therapy. Therefore, base the initial diabetes meal plan on the patient's appetite to restore or maintain appropriate body weight and allow for normal growth and development. Once the initial meal plan has been established, monitor weight, blood pressure, glycated hemoglobin A1c (A1C), lipids, and other clinical parameters to determine whether further modifications are needed to meet goals.

For individuals using either multiple-dose insulin (MDI) or continuous subcutaneous insulin infusion (CSII), lifestyle flexibility and maintaining optimal blood glucose control are achieved by developing personal algorithms that take into account the interplay of insulin, food intake, and physical activity. Using these algorithms, patients are able to systematically adjust insulin therapy as needed in response to deviations from usual patterns.[2]

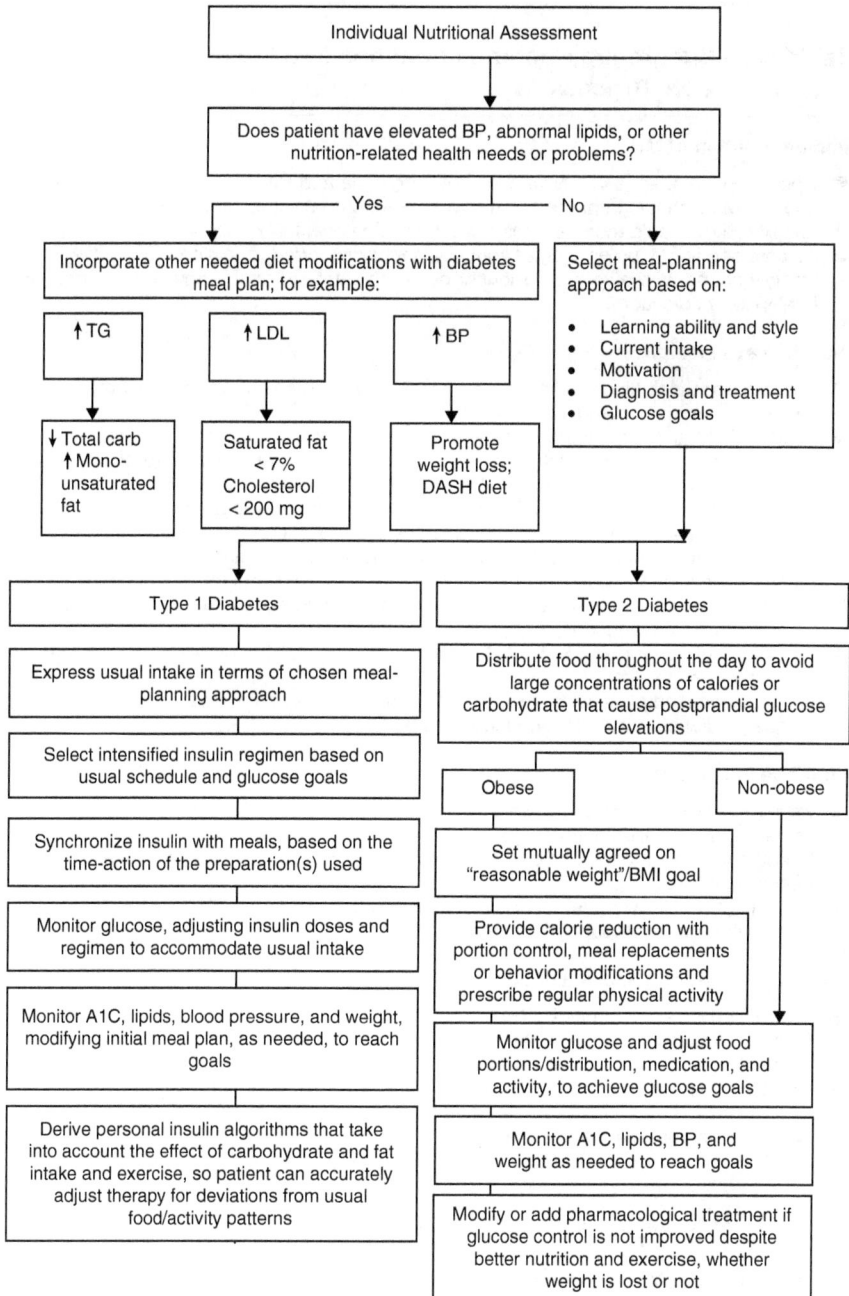

```
┌─────────────────────────────────────────────┐
│        Individual Nutritional Assessment      │
└─────────────────────────────────────────────┘
                      │
                      ▼
┌─────────────────────────────────────────────┐
│ Does patient have elevated BP, abnormal      │
│ lipids, or other nutrition-related health     │
│ needs or problems?                            │
└─────────────────────────────────────────────┘
        Yes                    No
```

Individual Nutritional Assessment

Does patient have elevated BP, abnormal lipids, or other nutrition-related health needs or problems?

Yes — No

Incorporate other needed diet modifications with diabetes meal plan; for example:

↑TG   ↑LDL   ↑BP

↓Total carb ↑Mono-unsaturated fat

Saturated fat < 7% Cholesterol < 200 mg

Promote weight loss; DASH diet

Select meal-planning approach based on:
- Learning ability and style
- Current intake
- Motivation
- Diagnosis and treatment
- Glucose goals

Type 1 Diabetes

Express usual intake in terms of chosen meal-planning approach

Select intensified insulin regimen based on usual schedule and glucose goals

Synchronize insulin with meals, based on the time-action of the preparation(s) used

Monitor glucose, adjusting insulin doses and regimen to accommodate usual intake

Monitor A1C, lipids, blood pressure, and weight, modifying initial meal plan, as needed, to reach goals

Derive personal insulin algorithms that take into account the effect of carbohydrate and fat intake and exercise, so patient can accurately adjust therapy for deviations from usual food/activity patterns

Type 2 Diabetes

Distribute food throughout the day to avoid large concentrations of calories or carbohydrate that cause postprandial glucose elevations

Obese   Non-obese

Set mutually agreed on "reasonable weight"/BMI goal

Provide calorie reduction with portion control, meal replacements or behavior modifications and prescribe regular physical activity

Monitor glucose and adjust food portions/distribution, medication, and activity, to achieve glucose goals

Monitor A1C, lipids, BP, and weight as needed to reach goals

Modify or add pharmacological treatment if glucose control is not improved despite better nutrition and exercise, whether weight is lost or not

BP, blood pressure; TG, triglycerides; LDL, low density lipoprotein; DASH, Dietary Approaches to Stop Hypertension

Figure 9.1—Nutrition management flow chart (updated).

Table 9.4—Integrating Recommendations into the Nutrition Care Process

Implementation of MNT

- Upon diagnosis, an RD/RDN who is knowledgeable and skilled in providing diabetes-specific MNT should implement three to six encounters within 6 months.
- The RD/RDN should then determine whether additional MNT encounters are needed.
- At least one follow-up encounter annually is recommended to reinforce education or lifestyle changes, evaluate and monitor outcomes, and determine any need for change in MNT or medications.

Nutrition assessment

- Client history, including medication and nutritional supplement history, past medical history, family history, and social history
- Food and nutrition history, including food intake (composition, adequacy, meal or snack patterns, environmental cues to eating, tolerance, current diets or food modifications); nutrition health awareness and management (knowledge and beliefs about nutrition recommendations, self-monitoring and management practices, prior education); physical activity and exercise (functional status, activity patterns, sedentary time, exercise intensity, frequency, and duration); and food availability (food planning, purchasing, preparation abilities and limitations; food safety; food program utilization; food insecurity)
- Biochemical data, medical tests, and procedures, including laboratory data (A1C, lipid profile, kidney function)
- Anthropometric measurements, including height, weight, BMI, growth rate, and rate of weight change
- Nutrition-focused physical finders, including general physical appearance, body language, digestive system, and blood pressure

Nutrition intervention

- Implement MNT, selecting from a variety of nutrition interventions to help patients achieve individualized nutrition goals.
- Encourage consumption of macronutrients based on dietary reference intakes for healthy children and adults.
- Implement nutrition education and counseling with emphasis on recommendations from major and contributing factors to nutrition therapy.

Nutrition monitoring and evaluation

- Coordinate care with multidisciplinary team.
- Monitor and evaluate food intake, medication, metabolic control, anthropometric measurements, and physical activity.
- Use blood glucose monitoring results to evaluate achievement of goals and effectiveness of MNT. Glucose monitoring results can help determine whether food or medication need to be adjusted.

Two different approaches can be used when a patient initiates intensive diabetes management. The first approach is a fixed carbohydrate and insulin plan, which involves prescribing a consistent carbohydrate meal plan based on the patient's usual intake and nutrition requirements. Prandial insulin dosages are then adjusted to the amount of carbohydrate in each meal to achieve target glycemia levels. Once the optimal insulin dosage for each meal is established, the insulin dose is "fixed." Education around the amount of carbohydrate in different foods should be provided so that the source of carbohydrate (e.g., fruit versus dairy versus grains) can be varied without changing the total carbohydrate content of the meal or snack.[1]

For patients who are skilled in carbohydrate counting and desire the flexibility of eating varying amounts of carbohydrate, a second approach is useful, namely, a flexible carbohydrate and insulin plan. This approach prescribes an insulin dose per quantity of carbohydrate (insulin-to-carbohydrate ratio [ICR]), so that the prandial insulin dose can be adjusted based on the desired amount of carbohydrate in the meal. For example, if a patient has an ICR of 1:10 g and wants to eat 50 g carbohydrate, they will then require 5 units of insulin (50 divided by 10). This approach allows patients more flexibility with food choices and quantities. The ICR can be determined by several methods but the most common are based on experience or the Rule of 500; for other methods see Table 9.8. Based on experience, if a patient consistently eats a lunch containing about 72 g carbohydrate and requires 8 units rapid-acting insulin when the pre-lunch blood glucose level is at target, this patient requires 1 unit insulin for every 9 g carbohydrate at lunch (72 divided by 8).[1] The rule of 500 (500 divided by total daily dose of insulin [TDD]) is also often used to find a starting point for the ICR. Similarly, it provides an estimate of how many grams of carbohydrate, 1 unit insulin covers. For example, a patient whose TDD dose is 50 units would divide 500 by 50 to achieve a ratio of 1:10. This ratio then may need to be adjusted (fine-tuned) based on an evaluation of postprandial blood glucose levels and food records. It is common for patients to have different ICRs for different meals.[6]

These meal-planning strategies arise from a strong scientific and behavioral base and describe a much less prescriptive approach than has commonly been used in the past. They acknowledge the difficulty in changing ingrained food habits, the wide range of diets that can be compatible with good diabetes control, and the importance of prioritizing the patient's preferences and lifestyle values while supporting increased flexibility and patient choice to the overall plan of care. Like other aspects of intensified management, they require more time and skill on the part of healthcare providers and patients than do simpler approaches that were widely used in the past.

STRATEGIES FOR TYPE 2 DIABETES

For patients with T2D, the primary focus of MNT is to promote healthful eating patterns that stress nutrient-dense foods in appropriate portions to attain and sustain body weight, glycemic, lipid, and blood pressure goals. In addition, MNT aims to prevent or delay risk of chronic complications, especially cardiovascular disease. While aiming to achieve and reach these goals, it is important to take into account an individual's food preferences, cultural preferences, literacy, access to healthful food, numeracy, eagerness to make behavioral changes, and barriers to change.[7] Near-normal blood glucose control reduces insulin resistance and preserves insulin secretory capacity in T2D. Eating plans that result in an energy deficit and modest weight loss (≥5% of body weight) often improve glycemic control and insulin resistance in the short term and, if maintained, can contribute to long-term improvements in the glycemic control of T2D.[8] The cutoff of 5% weight loss is the threshold needed for therapeutic benefit in T2D, including meaningful reductions in blood glucose, A1C, and triglycerides. The greater the weight loss (≥15% body weight), the greater the benefits, including reductions in the need for medications for blood pressure, lipids, and blood glucose.[2] For patients who are at risk of T2D, intensive lifestyle interventions that result in 7–10% weight loss are recommended. The risk of comorbidity increases with BMI in the overweight range and higher. Waist circumference is used as a measure of visceral fat. A waist circumference of ≥35 inches in women and ≥40 inches in men is used in conjunction with BMI to assess the risk of cardiovascular disease as well as the risk for T2D.

A structured, intensive lifestyle program that focuses on dietary changes, physical activity, behavioral strategies, and frequent contact with healthcare providers is a requirement to achieve and maintain a ≥5% weight loss. Such interventions aim to produce an energy deficit of 500–750 kcal/day and are modeled after the Diabetes Prevention Program (DPP). A DPP-based program aims for ≥16 sessions in 6 months and is intended as a long-term, thorough weight-loss program. Physical activity alone has only a modest effect on weight loss, but nevertheless it is important for improving insulin sensitivity, lowering blood glucose levels, and maintaining long-term weight loss. In order to achieve long-term maintenance, it is important to create eating plans that result in calorie reductions but also incorporate the patient's preferences and resources. Continued support and follow-up are essential for weight maintenance.[2]

Evidence suggests there is a not a "one-size-fits-all" eating pattern for all individuals with T2D, and meal planning should be individualized. One of the goals of MNT is to maintain the joy of eating and to present data in an open-minded manner, only limiting foods based on scientific evidence. Given the lack of evidence in favor of one specific eating pattern, key factors to focus on are: *1)* emphasis on nonstarchy vegetables, *2)* choosing whole foods versus highly processed foods, and 3) limiting added sugars and refined grains. Reducing carbohydrates improves blood glucose and can be integrated in a variety of eating patterns. Low-carbohydrate and very-low-carbohydrate (VLC) eating have been studied extensively in individuals with T2D. Evidence suggests that VLC diets, in the short term, may result in more weight loss than low-fat diets. In the longer term, however, differences in weight loss between VLC and low-fat diets are not significant, and weight loss is modest with both dietary approaches. The long-term effects of VLC diets are unknown; these diets may be deficient in fiber, vitamins, and minerals and usually rate low on palatability, thus making them difficult to sustain for a long period of time. A moderate reduction in carbohydrate can be considered for people with T2D and may be more efficacious.[7]

The Mediterranean-style, low-carbohydrate, vegetarian, or plant-based eating patterns are all examples of healthful eating patterns that have been reported to benefit individuals with T2D, but it is key to individualize the eating pattern to a patient's goals, needs, and personal preferences. Although the Mediterranean-style eating plan has shown potential for T2D remission and improved glycemic control, results have been mixed in a number of randomized controlled trials (RCTs). In an RCT by Esposito et al., patients on a low-carbohydrate Mediterranean-style eating plan had higher rates of partial diabetes remission versus those on a low-fat eating plan.[9] The PREDIMED trial compared a Mediterranean-style eating pattern with a low-fat eating pattern; after 4 years, subjects on the Mediterranean-style eating pattern had improved glycemic control, used fewer glucose-lowering medications, and had a lowered incidence of cardiovascular disease.[2] In the Dietary Intervention Randomized Controlled Trial (DIRECT), patients with T2D and obesity were randomized to low-carbohydrate, calorie-restricted lower-fat, and calorie-restricted Mediterranean-style eating patterns. The low-carbohydrate group had the lowest A1C, whereas the Mediterranean-style eating pattern group produced the lowest fasting plasma glucose.[2]

Eating plans that aim to achieve >5% weight loss in a short period of time (<3 months) can include meal replacements and VLC diets . VLC diets (providing ≤800 calories/day) and meal replacements should be considered for selected patients under the guidance of a medical provider with close monitoring. Meal replacements, typically consisting of shakes or prepackaged meals, can be safely used for one or two meals per day. They provide a defined amount of calories and nutrients and can result in significant weight loss. Use of meal replacements generally must be continued, however, to sustain the weight loss. Weight regain is typically greater in VLC diet eating plans versus intensive lifestyle modifications. If a VLC diet is considered, it must be part of a structured program that provides ongoing support.[5]

Weight-loss medications have been used in combination with lifestyle changes to successfully promote weight loss (5–10%) among individuals with T2D and overweight or obesity. Pharmacological therapy for obesity should be used only in patients with a BMI ≥27 kg/m². Metabolic surgery, which includes partial gastrectomies and bariatric procedures, promote effective weight loss and result in substantial improvement in glycemia and cardiovascular risk factors. Metabolic surgery results in superior weight loss, glycemic control, and reduction in cardiovascular risk factors compared to lifestyle or medical interventions. Metabolic surgery should be recommended as an option to treat patients with T2D and a BMI ≥40 kg/m² (BMI ≥37.5 kg/m² in Asian Americans) and patients with T2D and BMI ≥35–39.9 kg/m² (BMI ≥32.5–37.4 kg/m² in Asian Americans) who have not been able to maintain weight loss or have not had improvement in comorbidities with nonsurgical options. Metabolic surgery is an effective long-term treatment for diabetes. Diabetes remission postsurgery can range from 23% to 60% depending on the severity and duration of the diabetes prior to surgery.[10] With or without diabetes remission, patients with diabetes who underwent metabolic surgery maintained significant improvements in glycemic control for 5–15 years. The safety of metabolic surgery has significantly increased, especially with minimally invasive laparoscopic surgery. Mortality rates are 0.1–0.5%, comparable to surgeries such as cholecystectomies or hysterectomies. Major complications compare favorably to other elective surgeries. Metabolic surgery should be performed in a high-volume center with a multidisciplinary care team that can provide long-term support.[5]

The following strategies form the basis for dietary intervention in all people with T2D. When applied in conjunction with active monitoring of glucose, they also delineate the MNT component of intensified management for this group.

- The nutrition prescription should be based on lifestyle changes that patients are willing and able to make.
- Review the patient's usual intake with respect to total energy, food, and carbohydrate distribution throughout the day, fat intake (type and amount), and food selection.
- Distribute food throughout the day to eliminate large concentrations of calories or carbohydrate that may contribute to postprandial glucose elevation.
- Make recommendations regarding improvements in food choices to create a nutritionally adequate meal plan with reduced total, saturated, and trans fat, if needed.
- Advise patients regarding cholesterol intake per guidelines (see Table 9.3).
- If the patient is overweight, recommend an energy-deficit diet and regular physical activity to help promote modest, gradual weight loss of ≥5%. Significant weight loss can be promoted by a 500–750 kcal/day energy deficit.
- Monitor blood glucose and adjust food distribution, portions, and selection (as needed) in concert with medications and physical activity to achieve glucose goals.
- Monitor weight, blood pressure, A1C, lipids, and other clinical parameters, and modify the initial meal plan as needed to meet goals.

Traditionally defined "desirable" or "ideal" body weight is no longer used in setting weight goals for patients with diabetes. The guideline terminology "reasonable weight" refers to the weight an individual and his or her healthcare provider agree can be achieved and maintained, in both the short and long term. In addition, goals for BMI and waist circumference, mutually agreed on by the patient and practitioner, may be more achievable and realistic than focusing on a predetermined body weight goal.

MNT is not static and should be reassessed and modified with time. Patients may start with one eating plan and over time change or incorporate other eating plans to meet metabolic goals, personal preferences and changes in needs. While formulating plans, it is important to evaluate patients for disordered eating, eating disorders, or disrupted eating patterns and address them appropriately.

GLUCOSE MONITORING AND THE NUTRITION PLAN

BLOOD GLUCOSE MONITORING

Use of the results of blood glucose monitoring plays an essential role in the nutrition aspects of intensive diabetes management. Blood glucose monitoring provides the feedback needed to fine-tune the meal plan in concert with physical activity, medications (if used), and other relevant factors.

When evaluated in relation to food records, blood glucose monitoring can be used to refine the dietary approach in various ways. Postprandial glucose values can guide modification of the basic meal plan or can be used to tailor the patient's ICR or insulin adjustment algorithm. Review of food records in conjunction with glucose results reveals the effect of various single foods and food combinations. Such information, when used as the basis for determining prandial insulin dosing, can increase the patient's flexibility in food choices while maintaining or improving glucose control. Some sample monitoring strategies that help to fine-tune nutritional care are outlined in Table 9.5.

For all patients with T1D or T2D, the primary goal of MNT is to establish a healthy eating plan using the principles of MNT previously described. If pre- or postprandial glucose values are not within the target range despite a healthy, balanced diet, it may be prudent to commence or adjust an oral medication, incretin mimetic, or insulin. Fig. 9.1 illustrates schematically the process of nutrition intervention in intensive management, including the essential role of blood glucose monitoring in evaluating and adjusting intervention.

CONTINUOUS GLUCOSE MONITORING

CGM systems use a subcutaneous glucose sensor to continually measure interstitial glucose concentrations. These values correlate with plasma glucose levels, and these systems provide detailed information on glucose patterns and trends, including postprandial glucose values that are difficult to ascertain by episodic monitoring of blood glucose concentrations. They also provide information on the direction and rate of change of glucose concentrations. By allowing patients to observe glucose values and trends as they occur, CGM provides the patient with the opportunity to make decisions based on real-time glucose values and perform more timely therapy adjustments. There are two types of CGM systems, real-time CGM and intermittently scanned CGM. Although they both provide similar information regarding glucose trends, real-time CGMs will display glucose readings at all times and also provide alarms and alerts for glucose levels out of target range and rate of glucose change. Intermittently scanned CGM requires the patient to scan the sensor with their reader to observe the glucose readings and do not allow for real-time alarms or alerts. More detailed information on CGM is included in Chapter 7.

The data obtained from CGM allow for greater precision in matching the dose and timing of mealtime insulin to postprandial glucose profiles. CGM can be especially helpful for adjusting the insulin dose for meals that produce complex postmeal glucose profiles (e.g., pizza). CGM can be used to identify a problematic postmeal glucose pattern and then to monitor the postprandial pattern following various corrective bolusing schemes. In this way, the optimal dose and time parameters for the meal bolus can be determined.

CGM data can be an important tool for reshaping eating behavior because patients receive immediate feedback on their personal glycemic responses to their food choices. CGM has made it possible for users to more clearly see that the food factors that determine the postprandial glucose profile include not only the amount of carbohydrate but also the type of carbohydrate (i.e., glycemic index value) and the effect of fat, protein, caffeine, and alcohol. Foods with a high glycemic index may cause a postprandial glucose spike because of a mismatch between the rapid absorption of the carbohydrate and the less rapid onset of action of the

Table 9.5—Using Blood Glucose Monitoring to Fine-Tune Nutrition Therapy

Type of diabetes	Pharmacological management	Blood glucose monitoring schedule	Question to ask	Strategy to correct elevated blood glucose
T2D with obesity	None; oral diabetes medication(s), incretin mimetic, or insulin	Fasting	Does the overnight insulin or other oral glucose-lowering agent suppress hepatic glucose output sufficiently to produce desired fasting blood glucose level?	Reduce total calories; review bedtime snack and any other foods eaten overnight. Evaluate pharmacological management.
		2- to 4-h postprandial or next premeal blood glucose	Does available insulin (endogenous or exogenous) cover the meal eaten, producing the desire post-prandial value?	Reduce calories or carbohydrate and fat in meal. When obesity is present, food reduction and increased physical activity are preferred to increases in medication whenever possible. Consider the glycemic impact of carbohydrate ingested.
T1D or T2D nonobese	Insulin	Fasting	Does overnight exogenous insulin suppress hepatic glucose output sufficiently to produce desired fasting blood glucose level?	Adjust dose or timing of overnight insulin; review evening meal, bedtime snack, and any other foods eaten overnight. Consider adding another oral glucose-lowering agent or an incretin mimetic in patients with T2D. Insulin coverage may be needed for bedtime snack in those patients on CSII or MDI therapy.
		2- to 4-h postprandial (rapid-acting insulin analog) or next premeal value (regular insulin)	Is the premeal insulin dose appropriate?	Adjust dose or timing of premeal insulin; fine-tune patient's insulin algorithm; evaluate impact of quantity of carbohydrate (and glycemic impact [GI/GL]) of carbohydrate), protein, or fat consumed.
		Premeal (CSII or MDI only)	Is the basal insulin dose or rate (for CSII) correct?	Adjust basal insulin to bring premeal blood glucose into target range.

CSII, continuous subcutaneous insulin infusion; MDI, multiple-dose injection; GI/GL, glycemic index/glycemic load.

insulin bolus. Protein can increase postprandial glucose levels through increased hepatic glucose output, although it is usually a delayed effect seen ~1.5 h after the meal. Fat can affect postprandial glucose levels by slowing gastric emptying, thereby delaying the increase in postmeal glucose levels, and also by decreasing postprandial insulin sensitivity, leading to higher postmeal glucose levels than would be produced by a carbohydrate-equivalent low-fat meal. Caffeine, like fat, can reduce insulin sensitivity in some people, also leading to higher glucose levels. Alcohol has a glucose-lowering effect because it blocks glucose release from the liver. Alcoholic beverages containing significant carbohydrate initially may cause an increase followed by a later decrease in glucose levels. The multiplicity of food factors affecting postprandial glucose levels can make diabetes control challenging for the patient. By providing feedback on glycemic responses to various food factors, CGM can enable the motivated patient to improve glycemic control with less frequent hypoglycemia.[11]

HYPOGLYCEMIA

Nutrition strategies are important for the prevention of hypoglycemia in all people whose diabetes treatment includes insulin or an insulin secretagogue. Common nutrition factors that contribute to hypoglycemia risk are listed in Table 9.6; issues and strategies relative to each factor are discussed in the following sections.

OMITTING OR DELAYING PLANNED MEALS OR SNACKS

The risk of hypoglycemia from omitting or delaying meals is greatest in patients who use insulin regimens that include intermediate- and short-acting (regular) insulin. The increased risk is attributable to high circulating insulin levels between meals and overnight owing to the time–action profiles of intermediate- and short-acting insulin.[12] The risk of hypoglycemia also may be high if meals or snacks are omitted or delayed in patients using MDI regimens or in patients using an insulin secretagogue. Patients whose diabetes is treated by diet alone or those who use noninsulin therapies such as biguanides, pioglitazone, glucagon-like peptide 1 receptor agonists (GLP1-RA), dipeptidyl peptidase-4 inhibitors (DPP-4) or

Table 9.6—Nutrition Factors Contributing to Hypoglycemia

- Omitting or delaying planned meals or snacks
- Inappropriate timing of meals relative to insulin
- Imbalance between food and meal-related insulin dose because of
  - Inaccurate estimation of carbohydrate intake when calculating meal-related boluses
  - Consuming less carbohydrate than usual without adjusting insulin dose
- Inadequate carbohydrate supplementation for physical activity
- Consuming alcohol without food (or without adjusting insulin dose)
- Delayed absorption of carbohydrate when eating high-fat or low-glycemic-index meals and using a rapid-acting insulin analog

sodium–glucose cotransporter 2 (SGLT2) inhibitors as monotherapy are not at increased risk of hypoglycemia when meals are delayed or omitted.[13]

The risk for hypoglycemia should be considered when selecting a pharmacological regimen. Individuals whose work or other activities make it difficult to predict or control meal times will have less frequent hypoglycemia using noninsulin-based regimens that minimize hypoglycemia or, if needed, insulin regimens that allow more mealtime flexibility.[14]

All patients whose diabetes treatment includes insulin or an insulin secretagogue should receive education regarding appropriate meal timing for their particular regimen. Carrying a source of rapidly absorbed carbohydrate is a vital self-management behavior for all such patients to prevent hypoglycemia, particularly when meals are unavoidably delayed.[14]

INAPPROPRIATE TIMING OF INSULIN RELATIVE TO MEALS

The risk for hypoglycemia is greatest when the peak action of insulin is not synchronized with the peak of glucose entry into the bloodstream after a meal. Consider the following common scenario: the patient takes a bolus of short-acting insulin immediately before eating. Hyperglycemia occurs in the immediate postprandial period because carbohydrate is absorbed but insulin has not yet reached its peak action. Two to three hours later, when little or no carbohydrate is entering the circulation and insulin action has reached its peak, blood glucose levels decrease and hypoglycemia may occur. When using short-acting regular insulin, it is recommended to inject the insulin 30 min before a meal to better match insulin action and postprandial glucose availability. Rapid-acting insulin analogs, which achieve their peak action earlier than regular insulin, shorten the interval between administering the bolus and eating the meal. The shorter total duration of action of these insulins also reduces the risk for between-meal and nocturnal hypoglycemia (see Chapter 6, Multicomponent Insulin Regimens, for more detail). Blood glucose monitoring should be used to confirm optional insulin timing relative to meals because the action profiles of specific insulin preparations vary considerably from person to person and also are affected by injection site, exercise, and other factors.

In addition to modifying insulin administration or meal timing, another strategy to reduce the risk for hypoglycemia between meals is to include snacks in the meal plan. Snacks often are needed to prevent hypoglycemia in individuals using premixed insulins (see Chapter 6) because of the broad peak action curves of short-acting and intermediate-acting insulin (NPH insulin). The need for snacks often can be eliminated by using rapid-acting insulin analogs alone in CSII or in combination with a long-acting insulin, either glargine, detemir, or degludec, to provide between-meal insulin coverage.

IMBALANCE BETWEEN FOOD AND MEAL-RELATED INSULIN DOSE

Hypoglycemia may result when the meal-related insulin dose is too large relative to the amount of food eaten. In the intensively managed MDI or CSII patient who adjusts premeal boluses for anticipated intake, hypoglycemia most often occurs because of errors in estimating food or carbohydrate intake. Bolus calculations can be based on carbohydrate choices, carbohydrate intake, or known meal composition (menus), but irrespective of the method used, the algorithm used must be individualized to the patient. Many people benefit from a period of weighing and measuring their food to train their eye to accurately estimate portion sizes.

Unless the blood glucose level is decreasing rapidly, the meal insulin bolus should be given before starting the meal. In special circumstances, it may be advisable to inject the meal bolus at the end of a meal. Doing so allows more calibration of the bolus to the actual amount eaten and is particularly helpful in the management of young children with diabetes with unpredictable eating habits and during illness or pregnancy, when nausea may interfere with eating.

For patients on a fixed insulin plan, a fixed meal plan is required. If one parameter changes, the other must reflect this change. Although not all patients will choose to increase insulin doses to accommodate extra food intake—perhaps as a means of weight management—they should at least be given instruction on how to prevent hypoglycemia if a smaller-than-normal meal is eaten. Individual guidelines for insulin reduction could be used, or the missing carbohydrate could be replaced with another equivalent carbohydrate source such as fruit or a snack.

INADEQUATE FOOD SUPPLEMENTATION FOR EXERCISE

Blood glucose monitoring is required to calibrate insulin doses or carbohydrate intake to reduce hypoglycemia risk with exercise. The decision whether to adjust food or insulin is determined by the individual's diabetes management goals and is affected by whether the exercise is planned. When exercise is planned, the dose of insulin acting during the period of physical activity can be reduced to minimize hypoglycemia risk (see Chapter 6). For example, if a patient is going to participate in prolonged aerobic exercise (>30 min) they may choose to reduce their pre-exercise prandial bolus by 30–50% up to 90 min before exercise. This may need to be further adjusted based on the intensity and duration of activity. Anaerobic exercise (resistance training) can be associated with better glucose stability or even a modest rise in some patients, therefore potentially not necessitating a decrease in insulin. CSII and automated insulin delivery systems offer more flexibility by temporarily adjusting basal insulin rates to reduce risk of hypoglycemia during exercise without the need for a snack. When practical, a basal reduction of 50–80% can be attempted well before exercise (60–90 min) to decrease hypoglycemia during exercise and also decrease post-exercise hyperglycemia.[15]

If exercise is not planned with sufficient time to permit insulin dose adjustment, additional carbohydrate usually is needed to prevent exercise-related hypoglycemia. Depending on the blood glucose level at the start of exercise, as well as the type (aerobic or anaerobic or mixed), intensity and duration of the activity, the extra carbohydrate may be taken before, during, or after exercise. In general, if blood glucose levels are <100 mg/dL before starting exercise, carbohydrate should be ingested before the activity begins. During exercise of moderate intensity, glucose uptake is increased by 2–3 mg/kg/min or ~8–13 g/h, which supports the general recommendation to add 15 g carbohydrate for every 30–60 min of activity exceeding the patient's usual level of physical activity. Patients will need personalized guidelines based on blood glucose monitoring to guide carbohydrate supplementation for exercise. When exercise has been intense or prolonged, the risk for hypoglycemia extends up to 24 h post exercise. Therefore, additional snacks may be needed in the hours after exercise, or before bedtime, when strenuous exercise has occurred in the afternoon or evening. In addition, reduction of the amount of insulin administered after particularly lengthy or intense exercise may be required.[16]

Exercise is a central component of overall diabetes management for individuals attempting to reach and maintain a reasonable body weight. It is obviously preferable to avoid increasing food intake to cover exercise in such individuals. To better support weight management and calorie restriction goals, exercise can be scheduled after meals when blood glucose levels are peaking. If exercising after meals is not possible, or if it does not prevent hypoglycemia, medication doses should be decreased to allow exercise to occur without having to increase food intake.

Automated insulin delivery systems may be activated by patients to more aggressively reduce insulin titration or suspend insulin delivery before hypoglycemia occurs (exercise modes). However, hypoglycemia may still occur depending on the amount of insulin on board at the time of exercise, types and durations of exercise.[17]

CONSUMING ALCOHOL ON AN EMPTY STOMACH

Alcohol inhibits gluconeogenesis, interferes with the counterregulatory response to insulin-induced hypoglycemia and may impair hypoglycemia awareness.[18] Alcohol, therefore, may place people with diabetes, especially those on insulin or insulin secretagogues, at risk of delayed hypoglycemia. If alcohol is consumed in the evening, there is an increased risk for patients on insulin or insulin secretagogues to develop nocturnal or fasting hypoglycemia.[2] If sweet wines, liqueurs, or drinks made with regular soda or fruit juices are consumed, the carbohydrate may need to be offset with insulin. This should be done cautiously, however, because of the hypoglycemia risk associated with alcohol. On the other hand, if patients consume alcohol such as dry wines, light beers, and drinks made with noncaloric mixers, insulin administration may not be necessary. However, it is prudent to recommended that patients eat food when drinking alcohol to avoid hypoglycemia. Checking the blood glucose level before going to sleep is a recommended safety precaution for patients who have been drinking alcohol. An extra bedtime snack or reduction in the dose of bedtime insulin may be necessary.[18]

Patients with T2D typically are insulin resistant and have less of a risk of alcohol-hypoglycemia, unless they are using insulin or an insulin secretagogue to manage their diabetes.

ORAL TREATMENT OF HYPOGLYCEMIA

Helping each patient develop a personally calibrated treatment plan for hypoglycemia is a valuable strategy to promote better blood glucose control. Overtreatment of hypoglycemia is common and often is caused by a lack of or inadequate advice on appropriate treatment of hypoglycemia. When the same "take 15–20 g of carbohydrate" advice is given to all patients, the result will be inadequate treatment in some and excessive treatment in others. The increase in blood glucose level produced by a given amount of carbohydrate varies from person to person, primarily as a result of differences in body size and insulin sensitivity. For example, a given quantity of carbohydrate generally will increase the blood glucose level more in a small person than it will in a larger person.

To develop an individual hypoglycemia treatment algorithm for a patient, begin with the estimate that each 5 g glucose increases blood glucose ~20 mg/dL (1.1 mmol/L; an approximate value for a 150-lb [69-kg] person). With subsequent blood glucose monitoring, fine-tune this value, based on the patient's response to given amounts of glucose. For example, suppose a 100-lb (45-kg) woman finds that her blood glucose level is 40 mg/dL (2.2 mmol/L), and she wants to increase her blood glucose level by ~60 mg/dL (3.3 mmol/L) to 100 mg/dL (5.6 mmol/L). If she treats the hypoglycemia with 15 g carbohydrate expecting that each 5 g carbohydrate will increase her blood glucose 20 mg/dL but instead her blood glucose increases to 145 mg/dL (8.0 mmol/L), this demonstrates that every 5 g glucose increases her blood glucose by 35 mg/dL. The patient then can calibrate treatment of a subsequent episode of hypoglycemia based on the current blood glucose concentration and a personal blood glucose target. Providing the patient with an algorithm can avoid a potential source of treatment error because it eliminates the patient's need to perform calculations in a hypoglycemic state.[16]

Virtually any nonfat source of carbohydrate (e.g., saltines, regular soda, fruit juice, nonfat milk) can be used to treat hypoglycemia; however, glucose is the most rapid-acting carbohydrate source. Commercially prepared products, such as glucose tablets and glucose gels, are higher in available glucose than other high-carbohydrate foods that contain sugars such as fructose that are of no benefit in raising blood glucose levels and further add to the calories consumed from the treatment of hypoglycemia. In addition, glucose tablets/gels offer the advantages of more precise glucose dosing and a more predictable glucose absorption. They also are more easily portable and unlikely to serve as a snack, so they are more likely to be available when hypoglycemia occurs.[16]

FACILITATING NUTRITION SELF-MANAGEMENT

Achieving optimal glycemic control requires that the patient successfully balance food intake, diabetes medications, and physical activity. Rigid or strict diets generally are not conducive to achieving glycemic control, as they are not individualized to the unique characteristics, preferences, and lifestyle of the patient. In addition, most people are unable to sustain a structured eating plan for any significant length of time. Each patient who uses an intensified management approach must receive the depth of education required to build nutrition self-management skills.[19]

As previously described, this process begins with a nutrition assessment to enable the RD/RDN to tailor MNT to each patient's unique circumstances. The ensuing education process progresses from the mutual identification of specific goals through appropriate stepwise intervention and is guided throughout by an evaluation of the patient's knowledge and skill, as well as by clinical parameters. These processes of assessment and education are similar for every patient regardless of the specific approach to diabetes meal planning used.

MEAL-PLANNING APPROACHES FOR INTENSIFIED
MANAGEMENT

Several distinct meal planning systems commonly are used in diabetes MNT. Each stresses a different factor (e.g., calories, portion control, food choices, fat, or carbohydrate content). The DCCT demonstrated that many different approaches to meal planning can be used successfully in intensive management regimens.[1] The four major types of diabetes meal planning systems and the benefits of each are summarized in Table 9.7. The choice of a specific meal planning approach should be based on a review of the patient's current intake and food choices, clinical goals, learning style, and desire for flexibility.

Always consider the amount of time necessary to teach various meal-planning approaches. Sufficient and effective patient education and support materials must be available. Similarly, all approaches entail a staged program of education, progressing from simple concepts of diabetes nutrition management to the more in-depth knowledge that supports nutrition self-management and informed decision-making. Therefore, different meal-planning systems may be utilized with one patient.

CARBOHYDRATE COUNTING

Carbohydrate counting is a meal-planning system that involves determining the amount of carbohydrate eaten at a meal or a snack because these foods have the greatest impact on postprandial glucose levels. Patients can learn to count grams of carbohydrate or carbohydrate choices or exchanges, where one choice or exchange is equivalent to 15 g carbohydrate. Basic carbohydrate-counting skills help patients understand carbohydrate portions and encourage patients to aim for consistent intake at meals and snacks. This meal-planning system can be an effective way to improve glycemic control and is typically more appropriate for patients with T2D or those on fixed insulin regimens.

Advanced carbohydrate-counting skills involve precisely counting the grams of carbohydrate in all meals and snacks. Patients are encouraged to read food labels, look up the carbohydrate content of food online or with mobile apps, measure portion sizes, and use an individualized ICR to calculate the meal insulin dose. There are several different methods to calculate the initial ratio of insulin needed for the amount of carbohydrate consumed (see Table 9.8 and Chapter 6).

For additional information on carbohydrate counting, please see reference 20.

ADJUSTING INSULIN FOR PROTEIN AND FAT

Emerging evidence from recent research indicates that, in addition to carbohydrate, fat and protein can significantly modulate postprandial glucose concentrations in individuals with T1D. It is now recommended that selected individuals who have mastered carbohydrate counting and are experiencing the glycemic impact of fat and protein should receive education and adjust their mealtime insulin accordingly.[13]

In the early postprandial period (first 2–3 h), dietary fat reduces the glycemic rise through delayed gastric emptying and can increase the potential for early

Table 9.7 – Benefits and Drawbacks of Major Types of Meal-Planning Systems

System type	Description	Benefits	Drawbacks
General guidelines	USDA Choose My Plate Guidelines; Dietary Guidelines for Americans	Easy to understand Good initial teaching tools Focus is on healthy food choices	Low emphasis on measuring portions complicates coordinating insulin doses with food
Menu planning	Written-out individual sample menus	Specific Simple to use Can guide food choices while patient learns more advanced concepts Can use patient's preferred and available foods	Lack of flexibility to respond to unusual circumstances Keeps decision-making in hands of caregiver instead of patient
Food choices	Lists groups of foods of similar nutritional content, indicating portions of each that can be substituted for one another to provide variety; accompanied by a meal pattern that indicates the number of servings to be eaten from each group at each meal	Includes portion control Facilitates calorie adjustment Supports meal-planning materials, such as food lists, recipes, and menus Multiple nutrition concerns can be incorporated into a single plan	Food choice concept is difficult for many to understand Time-consuming to teach Can be limiting and prescriptive, especially if inadequate education is provided Does not always correlate with portions listed on food labels
Counting	Systems that focus on counting amounts of given nutrients: common ones are carbohydrate counting for glucose control and fat counting for calorie control or weight management	Allows greatest flexibility in food choices Emphasis is on carefully quantifying food intake Simple to teach and apply because of single-topic focus Carbohydrate counting is most common method for matching insulin to food intake	Focuses on a single nutrient at a time rather than overall diet quality. Other nutrition concepts (e.g., healthy food choices, cardiovascular risk reduction) must be taught separately. Difficult for patients who have cognitive impairment or learning disability

USDA, U.S. Department of Agriculture.

Table 9.8—Options to Calculate the Insulin:Carbohydrate Ratio

Method 1: Patient data	The method relies on the patient recording detailed contextual data (ideally for at least 1 week) of pre- and postprandial blood glucose, carbohydrates consumed at meals and snacks, and administered bolus insulin. Review these records to determine the amount of insulin the patient used to cover the carbohydrates, resulting in postprandial glucose values within target.	Example: - Preprandial glucose within target range - Consumed 50 g carbohydrates - Injected 5 units lispro - Postprandial glucose within target range - 50 / 5 = 10 - ICR = 1:10
Method 2: Rule of 500	This is a widely used method. The patient's TDD is calculated. The TDD is divided by 500 to obtain the ICR.	Example: - Basal insulin = 25 units - Bolus insulin = 5 units at breakfast, 8 units at lunch, and 10 units at dinner 5 + 8 + 10 = 23 bolus units - TDD = 23 + 25 = 48 units - 500 / 48 = 10.4 (round to 10) - ICR = 1:10
Method 3: Weight and TDD	Using this method, the patient's weight (in pounds) is multiplied by 2.8 and then divided by TDD.	Example: - Weight = 170 lb - TDD = 48 - 170 × 2.8 / 48 = 9.9 (round to 10) - ICR = 1:10
Method 4: Using the correction factor (CF)	If the patient's correction or insulin sensitivity factor is already known, multiply the CF by 0.33.	Example: - CF = 30 - 30 × 0.33 = 9.9 (round to 10) - ICR = 1:10

hypoglycemia. Delayed gastric emptying can delay the peak postprandial glucose level. In the absence of sufficient insulin, meals containing a significant amount of dietary fat can cause substantial late postprandial hyperglycemia (>3 h) as acute insulin resistance and hepatic glucose output increase. High-fat meals can increase insulin requirements by more than twofold.[11]

Likewise, protein can significantly increase late postprandial glycemia, although the effects differ depending on whether carbohydrate is included in the meal. When protein and carbohydrate are eaten together (e.g., sandwich with meat filling), as little as 30 g of protein can cause a significant increase in glycemia, thereby increasing insulin requirements. However, for high-protein–low-carbohydrate meals (e.g., steak and salad), at least 75 g protein (equivalent to ~8 oz steak) is needed before a significant effect is seen. Indeed, 75 g protein alone has been shown to increase blood glucose levels to the same extent as 20 g carbohydrate without insulin. As with dietary fat, the effects of protein are delayed and typically are seen >1.5 h after the meal.

Whereas meals high in fat and protein require more insulin to control late-postprandial hyperglycemia than low-fat, low-protein meals with the same carbohydrate content, the actual amount of additional insulin and the insulin delivery pattern required for high-fat or high-protein meals is highly variable between patients. The type of dietary fat does not seem to be as important in terms of glycemic excursions. Recent studies have provided some guidance for individuals using insulin pump therapy suggesting a combo, extended, or dual-wave bolus extending over 2–2.5 h with as much as a 65% increased meal bolus, delivered in a 30/70% split, may be necessary.[21] Another more recent study reported that depending on the amount of dietary fat ingested, on average participants require incrementally increased amounts of dual-wave insulin at each bolus. More specifically, for 20 g fat ingested, an additional 6% insulin was required to be split 74/26% over 73 min; for 40 g fat, an additional 6% insulin split 63/37% over 75 min; and for 60 g fat, an additional 21% insulin split 49/51% over 105 min.[22]

Alternatively, patients using MDI may need to cover the initial carbohydrate portion of the meal with a preprandial injection of rapid-acting or ultra-rapid-acting insulin analog, aiming to cover the rapidly absorbed ingested carbohydrate with 30–50% of the total meal insulin and then follow up with another bolus 30–60 min after the meal to cover the remaining 50–70% insulin need expected to cover the slow glucose rise from the fat/protein component of the meal. In practice, it would be advisable to start with dose increases of 15–20% for high-protein and 30–35% for high-fat meals, accompanied by close monitoring and frequent reviews. Doses need to be individualized and should be titrated as needed.

These studies clearly demonstrate that modern prandial insulin dose calculations need to consider meal macronutrient composition over and above simple meal carbohydrate content. The traditional carbohydrate-centric approach to prandial insulin dosing assumes that only carbohydrate-containing foods and beverages impact postprandial glycemia. In order to optimize immediate and late postprandial glycemic excursions, future insulin dosing algorithms and strategies will need to be increasingly sophisticated and personalized to cover meals of varying macronutrient composition.[23]

WEIGHT GAIN ASSOCIATED WITH INTENSIVE MANAGEMENT

Weight gain may accompany intensive management as tighter blood glucose control is achieved, and it affects patients regardless of age or sex. Factors thought to be associated with weight gain are failure to compensate for calories no longer lost via glycosuria, consumption of extra calories to treat more frequent episodes of hypoglycemia, and repletion of body water or protein lost during a period of poor glucose control. In addition, patients on intensive therapy may find that they can consume a greater variety of foods without loss of glucose control and therefore experience the same result from overeating as the rest of the population.[24]

Table 9.9—Prevention of Weight Gain during Intensive Management

- Minimize medications that promote weight gain for those patients with overweight or obesity.
- Aim to achieve an energy deficit at initiation of intensive management.
- Eliminate snacks between meals.
- Treat hypoglycemia with measured amounts of glucose.
- Engage in physical activity as part of intensive management.
- Decrease insulin doses before exercise instead of snacking.
- In patients with T2D, consider the effects of antihyperglycemic pharmacotherapy on weight.
- Consider weight-loss medications as adjunct to diet, physical activity, and behavioral counseling in selected patients.

PREVENTION

Experience suggests that the following strategies may be helpful (see Table 9.9):

- **Minimize medications that promote weight gain.** Multiple agents used to treat diabetes such as insulin secretagogues, thiazolidinediones, and insulin can cause weight gain. When possible, it is important to minimize medications that cause weight gain and use agents that are either weight neutral or promote weight loss, such as metformin, α-glucosidase inhibitors, SGLT2 inhibitors, GLP1-RA, and amylin mimetics. Providers should also carefully review a patient's concomitant medications that may cause weight gain, such as antipsychotics, antidepressants, glucocorticoids, injectable progestins, and anticonvulsants, and if possible provide alternatives.[5]
- **Aim to achieve an energy deficit at initiation of intensive management for those patients with overweight or obesity.** Significant weight loss can be achieved with a 500–750 kcal/day energy deficit. This is approximately 1,200–1,500 kcal/day for women and 1,500–1,800 kcal/day for men. A minimum weight loss of 5% is recommended for all patients with prediabetes or diabetes who are overweight. It important to take into account the patient's motivation, life circumstances, health status, preferences, food availability, cultural circumstances, and willingness to implement lifestyle changes when creating an individualized eating plan.[5]
- **Eliminate snacks between meals.** Older human insulin regimens including intermediate-acting (NPH) or regular insulin often necessitated snacks between meals to avoid hypoglycemia. Newer long-acting insulin analogs and rapid-acting insulin analogs provide greater flexibility with less hypoglycemia and weight gain than older insulin regimens. The analog insulins may be more easily adjusted to eliminate the need for between-meal snacks and subsequently lead to reduced caloric intake.[13] For example, if patients consistently require snacks between meals to avoid hypoglycemia, the basal insulin dose may need to be reduced. Children and adolescents may need snacks to provide sufficient calories for normal growth and development. Many young children have a snack in the middle of the morning and in the afternoon, and may eat again

before going to bed. Older children and adolescents generally have an after-school snack and may or may not have a snack before bed.

■ **Treat hypoglycemia with glucose.** Treating hypoglycemia with foods that contain fat or protein in addition to carbohydrate slows the correction of hypoglycemia and leads to increased caloric intake. Therefore, patients should be urged to avoid treating hypoglycemia with common snack foods such as cheese and crackers or candy bars. The appropriate amount of carbohydrate, preferably in the form of glucose (see the section Oral Treatment of Hypoglycemia) should be consumed to correct hypoglycemia.

■ **Engage in physical activity as part of intensive management.** Physical activity includes all movement that increases energy use and is an important part of the care of patients with diabetes. The type and amount of exercise should be individualized. Current exercise recommendations for most adults with T1D and T2D are to aim for 150 min or more of moderate-intensity aerobic activity per week with no more than 2 consecutive days without activity. If patients participate in more vigorous-intensity or interval training, shorter intervals (75 min/week) may be sufficient. Resistance exercises are recommended 2–3 times per week. Older adults benefit from flexibility training, such as yoga or tai chi 2–3 times per week.[7]

■ **Decrease insulin doses for activity that exceeds daily routines.** Traditional dogma has taught patients to eat more when they exercise more than usual, a practice that makes weight control more difficult. With practice and judicious use of blood glucose monitoring, CGM, insulin pumps, and/or automated insulin delivery systems, patients can become skilled at reducing their usual insulin doses to offset the effect of additional exercise.

■ **Consider antihyperglycemic pharmacotherapies that promote weight loss.** As mentioned previously, multiple agents may promote weight loss. For example, SGCT2 inhibitors and GLP1-RA are particularly useful in this regard, especially given their added cardio-renal benefit. GLP1-RA monotherapy typically results in greater weight loss than SGLT2 inhibitors, although further weight loss may be induced by combining "weight-friendly" therapies. Body weight reduction may vary widely between different therapies, even within the same class. For example, body weight in SUSTAIN 1–3 was significantly reduced with semaglutide 0.5 mg (3.7–4.3 kg) and semaglutide 1.0 mg (4.5–6.1 kg) versus comparators (1.0–1.9 kg).[25] In the CANVAS trial, which investigated the effect of canagliflozin on important cardiovascular outcomes, the overall reduction in percentage body weight varied substantially over time compared with placebo, resulting in a greater weight reduction at 12 months (–2.77%) in comparison to 3 months (–1.72%).[26]

■ **Consider weight-loss medications as adjunct to diet, physical activity, and behavioral counseling in selected patients.** Nearly all weight-loss medications approved by the U.S. Food and Drug Administration have shown improvement in glycemic control in T2D and delay of progression to T2D in those with prediabetes. Weight-loss medications may help patients better adhere to low-calorie diets and lifestyle changes leading to less weight gain associated with intensive management. Providers must balance potential benefits of weight-loss medication versus potential risk.[5]

REFERENCES

1. Anderson EJ, Richardson M, Castle G, et al. Nutrition interventions for intensive therapy in the Diabetes Control and Complications Trial. The DCCT Research Group. *J Am Diet Assoc* 1993;93(7):768–772

2. Evert AB, Dennison M, Gardner CD, et al. Nutrition therapy for adults with diabetes or prediabetes: a consensus report. *Diabetes Care* 2019;42(5): 731–754

3. Thomas D, Elliott EJ. Low glycaemic index, or low glycaemic load, diets for diabetes mellitus. *Cochrane Database Syst Rev* 2009(1):CD006296

4. Bowman L, Mafham M, Wallendszus K, et al. Effects of n-3 fatty acid supplements in diabetes mellitus. *N Engl J Med* 2018;379(16):1540–1550

5. American Diabetes Association. 8. Obesity management for the treatment of type 2 diabetes: *Standards of Medical Care in Diabetes—2020. Diabetes Care* 2020;43(Suppl. 1):S89–S97

6. Gillespie SJ, Kulkarni KD, Daly AE. Using carbohydrate counting in diabetes clinical practice. *J Am Diet Assoc* 1998;98(8):897–905

7. American Diabetes Association. 5. Facilitating behavior change and well-being to improve health outcomes: *Standards of Medical Care in Diabetes—2020. Diabetes Care* 2020;43(Suppl. 1):S48–S65

8. Wing RR, Look AHEAD Research Group. Long-term effects of a lifestyle intervention on weight and cardiovascular risk factors in individuals with type 2 diabetes mellitus: four-year results of the Look AHEAD trial. *Arch Intern Med* 2010;170(17):1566–1575

9. Esposito K, Maiorino MI, Petrizzo M, Bellastella G, Giugliano D. The effects of a Mediterranean diet on the need for diabetes drugs and remission of newly diagnosed type 2 diabetes: follow-up of a randomized trial. *Diabetes Care* 2014;37(7):1824–1830

10. Schauer PR, Nor Hanipah Z, Rubino F. Metabolic surgery for treating type 2 diabetes mellitus: now supported by the world's leading diabetes organizations. *Cleve Clin J Med* 2017;84(7 Suppl. 1):S47–S56

11. Bell KJ, Smart CE, Steil GM, et al. Impact of fat, protein, and glycemic index on postprandial glucose control in type 1 diabetes: implications for intensive diabetes management in the continuous glucose monitoring era. *Diabetes Care* 2015;38(6):1008–1015

12. Rave K, Klein O, Frick AD, Becker RH. Advantage of premeal-injected insulin glulisine compared with regular human insulin in subjects with type 1 diabetes. *Diabetes Care* 2006;29(8):1812–1817

13. American Diabetes Association. 9. Pharmacologic approaches to glycemic treatment: *Standards of Medical Care in Diabetes—2020. Diabetes Care* 2020;43(Suppl. 1):S98–S110

14. Delahanty LM, Halford BN. The role of diet behaviors in achieving improved glycemic control in intensively treated patients in the Diabetes Control and Complications Trial. *Diabetes Care* 1993;16(11):1453–1458

15. Riddell MC, Gallen IW, Smart CE, et al. Exercise management in type 1 diabetes: a consensus statement. *Lancet Diabetes Endocrinol* 2017;5(5):377–390

16. Bantle JP, Wylie-Rosett J, Albright AL, et al. Nutrition recommendations and interventions for diabetes: a position statement of the American Diabetes Association. *Diabetes Care* 2008;31(Suppl. 1):S61–S78

17. Riddell MC, Pooni R, Fontana FY, Scott SN. Diabetes technology and exercise. *Endocrinol Metab Clin North Am* 2020;49(1):109–125

18. Tetzschner R, Nørgaard K, Ranjan A. Effects of alcohol on plasma glucose and prevention of alcohol-induced hypoglycemia in type 1 diabetes: a systematic review with GRADE. *Diabetes Metab Res Rev* 2018;34(3):e2965

19. Evert AB, Boucher JL, Cypress M, et al. Nutrition therapy recommendations for the management of adults with diabetes. *Diabetes Care* 2013;36(11): 3821–3842

20. Scheiner G. Counting carbohydrates like a pro. Practical tips for accurate counts. *Diabetes Self Manag* 2009;26(2):8, 10–12, 14

21. Bell KJ, Toschi E, Steil GM, Wolpert HA. Optimized mealtime insulin dosing for fat and protein in type 1 diabetes: application of a model-based approach to derive insulin doses for open-loop diabetes management. *Diabetes Care* 2016;39(9):1631–1634

22. Bell KJ, Fio CZ, Twigg S, et al. Amount and type of dietary fat, postprandial glycemia, and insulin requirements in type 1 diabetes: a randomized within-subject trial. *Diabetes Care* 2020;43(1):59–66

23. Evert AB. Factors beyond carbohydrate to consider when determining meantime insulin doses: protein, fat, timing, and technology. *Diabetes Spectr* 2020;33(2):149–155

24. The DCCT Research Group. Weight gain associated with intensive therapy in the Diabetes Control and Complications Trial. *Diabetes Care* 1988;11(7): 567–573

25. Fonseca VA, Capehorn MS, Garg SK, et al. Reductions in insulin resistance are mediated primarily via weight loss in subjects with type 2 diabetes on semaglutide. *J Clin Endocrinol Metab.* 2 April 2019 [Epub ahead of print]

26. Ohkuma T, Van Gaal L, Shaw W, et al. Clinical outcomes with canagliflozin according to baseline body mass index: results from post hoc analyses of the CANVAS program. *Diabetes Obes Metab* 2020;22(4):530–539

Index

Note: Page numbers followed by an *f* refer to figures. Page numbers followed by *t* refer to tables.